MOHS AND CUTANEOUS SURGERY

MOHS AND CUTANEOUS SURGERY

MAXIMIZING AESTHETIC OUTCOMES

Edited by

ALEXANDER BERLIN

Director of the DFW Skin Surgery Center in Arlington, Texas,
and
Assistant Clinical Professor of Dermatology,
Rutgers New Jersey Medical School,
Newark, New Jersey, USA

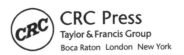

CRC Press
Taylor & Francis Group
Boca Raton London New York

CRC Press is an imprint of the
Taylor & Francis Group, an **informa** business

CRC Press
Taylor & Francis Group
6000 Broken Sound Parkway NW, Suite 300
Boca Raton, FL 33487-2742

First issued in paperback 2019

© 2015 by Taylor & Francis Group, LLC
CRC Press is an imprint of Taylor & Francis Group, an Informa business

ISBN-13: 978-1-4822-2136-7 (hbk)
ISBN-13: 978-0-367-37817-2 (pbk)

Visit the Taylor & Francis Web site at
http://www.taylorandfrancis.com

and the CRC Press Web site at
http://www.crcpress.com

CONTENTS

PREFACE

Achieving the best aesthetic results in Mohs and other cutaneous surgery requires proper patient selection and careful surgical technique, as well as meticulous postoperative care. However, despite the best efforts on the part of both surgeon and patient, complications may develop, sometimes resulting in suboptimal or objectionable scarring. This book deals with all aspects of putting forth the best effort to achieve the best aesthetic results in reconstructive skin surgery, as well as the numerous techniques available today for the correction of untoward healing.

Alexander L. Berlin

CONTRIBUTORS

Alexander L. Berlin, MD
DFW Skin Surgery Center, PLLC
Arlington, Texas

and

Division of Dermatology
New Jersey Medical School
Newark, New Jersey

Jeremy S. Bordeaux, MD, MPH
Department of Dermatology
University Hospitals Case Medical Center
Case Western Reserve University
Cleveland, Ohio

Christopher T. Burnett, MD
Dermatology Associates of Wisconsin
Milwaukee, Wisconsin

Sean Bury, MD
Division of Otolaryngology Head and
    Neck Surgery
Department of Surgery
George Washington University
Washington, DC

Lara K. Butler, MD
Department of Dermatology
Lahey Clinic Hospital
Harvard Medical School
Burlington, Massachusetts

Suneel Chilukuri, MD
Bellaire Dermatology Associates
Bellaire, Texas

and

Department of Dermatology and
    Dermatologic Surgery

Memorial Hermann F.P. Residency
    Program
Houston, Texas

and

Columbia University College of Physicians
    and Surgeons
New York, New York

and

Baylor College of Medicine
Houston, Texas

Joel L. Cohen, MD
AboutSkin Dermatology and
    DermSurgery
Englewood, Colorado

and

Department of Dermatology
University of Colorado
Aurora, Colorado

and

Department of Dermatology
University of California Irvine
Irvine, California

Brett Coldiron, MD
University of Cincinnati
Cincinnati, Ohio

Sarah J. Felton, MD
Consultant Dermatologist and
    Dermatological Surgeon
Oxford University Hospitals
Oxford, U.K.

Scott W. Fosko, MD
Department of Dermatology
Saint Louis University School of Medicine
Saint Louis, Missouri

Laura Kline, MD
Piedmont Plastic Surgery and
  Dermatology
Charlotte, North Carolina

Sailesh Konda, MD
Department of Dermatology
Loma Linda University Medical Center
Loma Linda, California

Matteo C. LoPiccolo, MD
Toledo Clinic Dermasurgery and Laser
  Center
Toledo, Ohio

and

Dermatology Specialists
Shelby, Mississippi

and

Department of Dermatology
Henry Ford Health System
Detroit, Michigan

Ian A. Maher, MD
Department of Dermatology
Saint Louis University
Saint Louis, Missouri

David M. Ozog, MD
Division of Mohs and Dermatological
  Surgery

Department of Dermatology
Henry Ford Hospital
Detroit, Michigan

Ali M. Rkein, MD
English Dermatology Centers
Gilbert, Arizona

Thomas E. Rohrer, MD
SkinCare Physicians
Chestnut Hill, Massachusetts

and

Department of Dermatology
Brown University School of Medicine
Providence, Rhode Island

Jordan B. Slutsky, MD
Division of Mohs Surgery and Cutaneous
  Oncology
Department of Dermatology
Stony Brook University Hospital
Stony Brook, New York

Divya Srivastava, MD
Department of Dermatology
UT Southwestern Medical Center
Dallas, Texas

Irene J. Vergilis, MD
Dermatology and Skin Surgery
New York, New York

and

Department of Dermatology
Rutgers University – Robert Wood
  Johnson Hospital
Somerset, New Jersey

PART I

Preoperative, Intraoperative, and Immediate Postoperative Period: Optimizing Surgical Outcomes

Chapter 1

Wound Healing and Surgical Planning

Alexander L. Berlin, Sarah J. Felton, Christopher T. Burnett, and Divya Srivastava

INTRODUCTION

In 1938, Frederic E. Mohs revolutionized surgical treatment of skin cancer, allowing for the precise localization and removal of tumor cells. When the use of the original escharotic paste was replaced by the fresh-frozen technique, same-day removal of cancer and subsequent repair of the surgical defect became possible.

As a tissue-sparing technique, Mohs surgery offers the possibility of the least resulting scarring. In the United States, dermatologic surgeons perform the majority of head and neck cutaneous reconstructions in the Medicare population, including flaps, grafts, and primary closures.[1] Therefore, Mohs surgeons are uniquely positioned to provide the most aesthetic results following complete tumor resection.

The route to achieving the best aesthetic outcome starts before tumor extirpation is undertaken, with appropriate surgical planning and understanding of the cutaneous wound healing process, both in the general population and in pathological states. It is to these issues that this introductory chapter will be devoted.

WOUND HEALING

Since the result of any cutaneous injury, including Mohs surgery, is a wound, it is very important to understand the process of wound healing. Though the specific molecular events underlying this process are still being worked out, it has become clear that complex interactions take place between various cell types, the extracellular matrix (ECM), and numerous released chemical mediators. Though they often overlap, it is helpful to organize the individual events involved in cutaneous wound healing into three traditionally recognized phases: inflammatory, proliferative, and remodeling. Though initial wound hemostasis is occasionally separated into its own "coagulation" phase, it will be discussed here as part of the inflammatory phase.

Inflammatory Phase

The inflammatory phase is composed of the vascular response and the cellular response. The initial physiological response to injury is the achievement of hemostasis and the formation of a provisional wound matrix.

Vascular Response   Immediately following injury to a blood vessel, platelets are activated by exposed collagen via glycoprotein Ia/IIa surface receptors.[2] Activated platelets release a variety of chemical mediators from their dense and alpha granules, including adenosine diphosphate (ADP), von Willebrand factor (vWF), thrombin, fibrinogen, transforming growth factor-β1 (TGF-β1), and several growth factors, such as platelet-derived growth factor (PDGF). vWF binds to collagen, as well as to vWF receptors on platelets, leading to platelet adhesion.[3,4] Both fibrinogen and vWF then bind to platelet glycoprotein IIb/IIIa receptors, resulting in platelet aggregation.[5,6] In addition, platelet activation induces membrane enzyme phospholipase A2. This results in the production of thromboxane A2 (TXA2), which causes vasoconstriction and further induces the expression of glycoprotein IIb/IIIa receptor.[7,8] Combined, these processes lead to the initial formation of a platelet plug, which may temporarily occlude a bleeding vessel.

Additionally, both the extrinsic and the intrinsic coagulation cascades are activated by contact with tissue factor in the injured skin and exposed fibrillar collagen, respectively. These ultimately lead to the formation of thrombin, a powerful platelet activator, which also converts fibrinogen to fibrin. Fibrin then acts as mortar between adherent platelets, leading to the formation of a fibrin clot. In addition to fibrin, the clot also contains fibronectin, thrombospondin, and other molecules, which form the initial scaffold for the influx of migrating cells.[9,10]

Platelets synthesize or store a variety of vasoactive, chemotactic, and proliferative mediators. Histamine is released by platelets and other cells and causes vasodilation and vascular permeability, allowing for cellular infiltration into the wound. PDGF has been shown to be chemotactic for neutrophils, macrophages, fibroblasts, and smooth muscle cells.[11,12] TGF-β1 is also chemotactic for fibroblasts, macrophages, and other cell types but, in addition, stimulates new collagen production.[13,14,15] Furthermore, together with endothelial cell selectin (E-selectin), platelet selectin (P-selectin) facilitates neutrophil margination, rolling, and capture, stimulating neutrophil influx.[16] Thus, platelet activation and aggregation directly contribute to the ensuing cellular response.

Cellular Response   In the early phase of the cellular response, neutrophils are recruited to the site of injury and typically persist for 2–5 days. As mentioned above, they are induced to infiltrate into the wound through the action of various chemotactic molecules, some of which are derived from platelets and other cells, while others may be released as a result of tissue damage (e.g., bradykinin and fibrin degradation products) or bacterial activation of the complement system (e.g., complement protein 5a). Through subsequent interactions between adhesion molecules on their surfaces and those on endothelial cells, neutrophils migrate out of blood vessels in the process of diapedesis.[17,18] Once in the wound, neutrophils phagocytose and kill bacteria through oxidative burst; additionally, they help to degrade matrix proteins and clear necrotic tissue.

In the late phase of the cellular response, monocytes are recruited from the circulation to enter the injury zone, thus becoming tissue macrophages. This typically begins around

3 days after cutaneous injury. Various chemotactic mediators of this influx have been identified; they may include PDGF, thrombin, TGF-β, and monocyte chemoattractant protein-1 (MCP-1).[19,20,21,22]

Macrophages are antigen-presenting cells critical to the wound healing process, and their dysfunction can lead to abnormal healing, including chronic wounds, ulcers, and hypertrophic scarring.[23] Similar to neutrophils, they also phagocytose and kill bacteria and eliminate debris. In addition, they clear residual neutrophils and other apoptotic cells; support fibroblast migration, proliferation, and differentiation; induce neovascularization; and promote ECM synthesis.[24] These functions are mediated through numerous potent growth factors synthesized and secreted by macrophages, including PDGF, basic fibroblast growth factor (bFGF), vascular endothelial growth factor (VEGF), TGF-α, and TGF-β.[25]

Animal models have demonstrated that selective ablation or deactivation of macrophages leads to decreased collagen deposition, angiogenesis, and cellular proliferation; loss of myofibroblast differentiation and wound contraction; and delayed reepithelialization.[26,27] In this way, macrophages provide a critical link to the next phase of the wound healing process, the proliferative phase.

Proliferative Phase

In the proliferative phase, cellular migration and proliferation predominate. The goal of this phase is to achieve the restoration of epidermal integrity through reepithelialization and that of dermal support through angiogenesis, fibroplasia, and ECM synthesis.

Reepithelialization   The process of reestablishment of the epidermis starts with keratinocyte migration from the wound edges and, in partial-thickness wounds, from skin appendages, such as the bulge region of the hair follicle.[28,29] This migration may be stimulated by the loss of contact inhibition, as well as through the release of numerous cytokines and growth factors, such as TGF-β, epidermal growth factor (EGF), and keratinocyte growth factor (KGF), and by macrophages, fibroblasts, and other cells.[30,31] Previously described hypotheses on keratinocyte migration include the "leapfrog" and the "train," or epidermal tongue extension, methods, though a recent three-dimensional *in vitro* model revealed a novel mechanism of reepithelialization: an extending shield.[32]

Keratinocytes near the wound edge develop pseudopod-like projections, lose their desmosomal and hemidesmosomal attachments, and reorganize their intracellular cytoskeletons, including actin filaments, in the direction of movement. This process is likely regulated by RhoGTPases, a family of small GTPases that include Rho, Rac, and Cdc42.[33] Activated keratinocytes also express collagenase-1, also known as matrix metalloproteinase-1 (MMP-1), which severs adhesions to collagen in the underlying dermal matrix, allowing migration until complete epidermal merging and reappearance of the basement membrane have been achieved.[34,35]

While migrating cells do not actively proliferate, trailing keratinocytes do, contributing to complete reepithelialization. This difference in behavior appears to be influenced by a number of growth factors and cytokines, such as EGF and TGF-β1.[36,37] Subsequently, keratinocyte differentiation leads to the restoration of epidermal barrier function. Expression of various mediators, such as KGF in fibroblasts and activin in basal keratinocytes, may affect epidermal redifferentiation.[38,39]

Angiogenesis   Angiogenesis, or neovascularization, in a healing wound is a complex process aimed at reestablishment of tissue perfusion in response to low-oxygen conditions. A vascular network may be formed *de novo* or as a result of anastomosis to existing blood vessels.

Similarly to the keratinocytes discussed above, endothelial cells near the wound edge undergo conformational changes and migrate into the healing wound along the fibrin/fibronectin network within the fibrin clot, thus forming capillary sprouts, or buds. Endothelial activating and chemotactic factors include lactic acid, bFGF, VEGF, TGF-β, angiopoietin, and mast cell tryptase, whereas thrombospondin inhibits migration, proliferation, and survival of endothelial cells.[40,41] Endothelial cells also release MMPs, allowing for their migration toward the angiogenic stimulus.[42]

The orientation of capillary sprouting is influenced by the interaction between the ECM and endothelial cell adhesion molecules (integrins). Furthermore, the expression of integrin receptors is affected by the surrounding ECM. As a result, fibrin and fibronectin stimulate integrin expression and support capillary sprouting, whereas collagen, as encountered in late granulation tissue, does not.[40] Capillary sprouts begin to interconnect, forming vessel loops and eventually differentiating into arterioles and venules. As discussed below, in the remodeling phase, blood vessels may undergo apoptosis when they are no longer needed for tissue perfusion.

Fibroplasia/Granulation Tissue Formation   In addition to the newly formed blood vessels, granulation tissue contains fibroblasts and their products: collagen and elastin fibers and ground substance. Fibroblasts migrate into the wound along the fibronectin scaffold and start proliferating in response to multiple factors, many of which are released by the activated macrophages, including PDGF, bFGF, and TGF-β1.[43,44] Additional chemotactic and proliferative factors may be released by mesenchymal stem cells migrating into the wound.[45]

Once in the wound, fibroblasts perform several functions. Some fibroblasts differentiate into myofibroblasts, cells primarily responsible for wound contraction through their abundance of actin and myosin filaments, as well as their interactions with the fibronectin fibrillar network.[46] This differentiation, as evidenced by the expression of α-smooth muscle actin (α-SMA), appears to be induced by many of the same factors that influence fibroblast influx and proliferation, including PDGF and TGF-β1.[47,48] It is unclear why only some populations of fibroblasts undergo this process, although a recent *in vitro* study indicated induced differentiation of fibroblasts that are in direct contact with neuronal processes.[49]

The main function of fibroblasts in a healing wound is the synthesis of components of the ECM, including collagen, glycosaminoglycans (GAGs) and proteoglycans, and elastin. This function is induced by several mediators, including TGF-β and connective tissue growth factor (CTGF).[50] CTGF itself is released by fibroblasts in response to macrophage-derived TGF-β1 and may act in an autocrine fashion to stimulate further chemotaxis and proliferation of fibroblasts, as well as new collagen production.[43,51,52] Fibrinogen matrix serves as the scaffold for new collagen deposition. Initially, fibroblasts preferentially synthesize type III, or fetal-like, collagen. Type III collagen exhibits a smaller fibril diameter and less cross-linking than type I collagen, the predominant type in adult skin.[53] Collagen type switching occurs later in the wound healing process, during remodeling, as discussed in the section "Remodeling Phase."

The ECM also contains GAGs and proteoglycans, the major components of ground substance. Hyaluronic acid, the first GAG to be synthesized in a healing wound, can store large amounts of extracellular water, contributing to tissue edema. Other GAGs, including chondroitin sulfate, dermatan sulfate, and heparin sulfate, form proteoglycans by attaching to a protein core after their synthesis by the fibroblasts. The resulting ground substance imparts supportive and protective functions to the dermis.

Remodeling Phase

During the remodeling phase, which can persist for 6–24 months, the dermal matrix continues to be deposited and modified. Collagen, ground substance, and fibronectin are synthesized and form a scaffold for the subsequent changes in the wound.

While the total amount of collagen continues to increase early in the wound healing process, an equilibrium is achieved in the remodeling phase, whereby the rate of collagen synthesis equals that of collagen degradation. At the same time, the tensile strength of the wound continues to increase, reaching approximately 10% that of uninjured skin by 1 week and 40% by 1 month but never exceeding 80% of the original strength. In addition, beginning at 1 week post–injury, wounds closed under tension exhibit greater tensile strength than tensionless wounds.[54,55] These changes are attributed to several factors, including variable expression of collagen types, greater collagen cross-linking, changes in the composition of other ECM components, and collagen fiber reorientation.

During remodeling, previously deposited type III collagen is degraded, mainly through the action of tissue collagenase-1 and -2 (also known as MMP-1 and -8), while type I collagen is synthesized in its place. As mentioned in the section "Fibroplasia/Granulation Tissue Formation," type I collagen fibrils are more extensively cross-linked than those of type III collagen. Cross-linking is accomplished by the action of lysyl oxidase on lysine and hydroxylysine residues.

Several signaling molecules may contribute to predominance of type I over type III collagen gene expression. For example, endothelin-1 (ET-1) and TGF-β isoforms 1 and 2 are associated with increased collagen type I deposition in adults, whereas wounds in fetal skin exhibit much higher levels of TGF-β3 than of the other two isoforms.[56,57,58] This process appears to be tightly controlled. Thus, excessive inhibition of MMPs by tissue inhibitors of metalloproteinases (TIMPs) and aberrations in the relative ratio of the two collagen types may lead to abnormal healing.[59,60,61]

Wound tension and stress appear to affect the orientation of collagen fibers, with those oriented parallel to the vector of tension appearing to be less susceptible to degradation by collagenases. This function is likely mediated by various adhesion molecules, such as fibroblast integrin receptors.[62,63] Additionally, other components of the ECM, including proteoglycans, decrease as the wound matures, leading to reduced extracellular water content. ECM degradation may be related at least in part to keratinocyte-induced dermal fibroblast expression of several MMPs.[64]

Initiated during the proliferative phase, wound contraction continues throughout the remodeling phase and is mediated mainly by myofibroblasts. This also appears to be related at least in part to mechanical tension from the surrounding ECM, which increases myosin expression.[65] Excessive myofibroblast activity may result in hypertrophic scarring and scar contracture;[66] conversely, recent evidence suggests that induction of myofibroblast apoptosis by recombinant bFGF may lead to scarless healing.[67]

While angiogenesis in an acutely healing wound has been researched extensively, blood vessel regression in the remodeling phase is still being worked out. A variety of antiangiogenic and apoptotic signals may be involved in this process and may be dependent on local oxygenation and perfusion, feedback mechanisms, and changing biomechanical properties of the ECM.[68]

As the remodeling phase progresses, the scar matures and eventually becomes largely acellular and avascular. Normally a tightly regulated process, cutaneous wound healing may be affected by a large variety of factors. Some may lead to delayed healing and chronic wounds, while others result in pathological scarring, such as keloid formation. We will now examine some of these factors as they pertain to dermatological surgery.

ROLE OF PATIENT FACTORS IN CUTANEOUS WOUND HEALING

While many factors cannot be predicted or planned for, some are commonly associated with delayed, prolonged, or otherwise poor wound healing and with resulting suboptimal cosmetic outcome. Of these, some are easily modifiable while others may be adjusted only slightly or not at all prior to surgery.

Diabetes

Impaired wound healing is a recognized complication of diabetes mellitus and is caused by any of a number of factors. Of particular importance are reduced migration and proliferation of both keratinocytes and fibroblasts and decreased angiogenesis during hyperglycemic states.[69] In addition, hyperglycemia impairs the immune response, so that sufferers are more prone to wound infections, which further inhibit healing.

Hemoglobin A1c (HbA$_{1c}$) reflects the degree of glycemic control over the preceding 2 to 3 months. Levels below 5.6% are considered normal, and for many diabetics, the goal is to maintain HbA$_{1c}$ levels between 6.5% and 7%. A study investigating healing rates in diabetic patients demonstrated a significant association between elevated HbA$_{1c}$ levels (over 7%) and prolonged wound healing.[70] It is therefore important to try to optimize glycemic control perioperatively and to plan surgery accordingly. Thus, second intent healing (also referred to as second intention or secondary intention healing) in a poorly controlled diabetic patient following Mohs surgery may not be the best option, as impaired granulation tissue formation may lead to a nonhealing ulcer.

Smoking

Nicotine and other constituents of tobacco smoke, such as carbon monoxide, tar, formaldehyde, and hydrogen cyanide, have detrimental effects on wound healing.[71] These effects are multifactorial; mechanisms may include decreased tissue oxygenation, altered collagen formation, and increased propensity for bacterial infection.[72] Studies have demonstrated a reduction in cutaneous blood flow after smoking a single cigarette, which could place random-pattern flaps and skin grafts in particular at risk for necrosis (Figure 1.1).[73,74] In addition, for all types of repairs, there is an increased risk for delayed healing and wound dehiscence in smokers.

Patients should therefore be counseled regarding smoking cessation. Ideally, patients would cease smoking well in advance of surgery (at least 2–4 weeks), with continued abstention during the postoperative period. However, this may not feasible for many patients, in particular the heaviest smokers, who are consequently at highest risk for complications. It should therefore be emphasized to patients that smoking should be reduced as much as possible to decrease this risk.

Nicotine replacement therapies avoid exposure to numerous toxic chemicals that are present in cigarette smoke. Transdermal nicotine replacement patches have been the subject of the most in-depth studies, but a general consensus as to their overall effects on wound healing has not been reached. A randomized controlled trial confirmed significant reduction in postoperative wound infections with smoking cessation, even with the use of nicotine replacement therapies.[75] However, concerns exist about the use of smokeless cigarettes, particularly due to their lack of regulation, the absence of peer-reviewed studies investigating their safety, and the high variation in the amount of vaporized nicotine they produce.

Alcohol Consumption

Alcohol exposure can impair several components of the wound healing process. *In vitro* ethanol exposure impairs collagen production in human fibroblasts and at high concentrations can limit fibroblast proliferation.[76,77] Similarly, *in vivo* studies have demonstrated diminished lysyl oxidase activity, decreased accumulation of collagen and hyaluronic acid, and lowered wound breaking threshold in mice exposed to ethanol.[76]

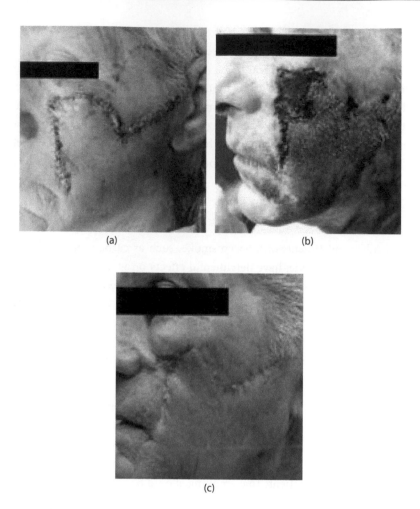

FIGURE 1.1   Flap necrosis in a heavy smoker (over three packs per day). (a) Immediate result following reconstruction. (b) Extensive flap necrosis at 1 week. Extensive ecchymosis was also present due to his antiplatelet therapy (aspirin and clopidogrel), but no hematoma occurred. (c) Final outcome after second intent healing.

Alcohol exposure also impairs several aspects of hemostasis, potentially leading to postoperative bleeding. Thrombocytopenia is known to occur in severe alcoholism; however, the platelet count trends upward within 2–5 days of alcohol cessation.[78] Several studies have demonstrated the ability of alcohol to inhibit platelet aggregation.[79,80] Alcohol intake has also been associated with higher fibrinolytic activity and decreased levels of coagulation factors.[81,82] Because of the potential adverse effects of impaired wound healing and bleeding, patients should avoid alcohol consumption in the pre- and postoperative periods to optimize the surgical outcome (Figure 1.2).

Immunosuppression

The incidence of nonmelanoma skin cancers, especially squamous cell carcinoma, is significantly increased in patients with a history of solid organ transplantation, because of

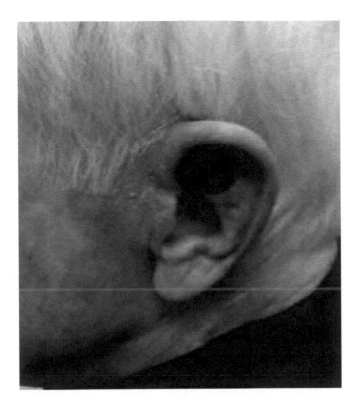

FIGURE 1.2   Graft necrosis in a patient who admitted to drinking alcohol in the early postoperative period, with resultant slow hemorrhage around the recipient site.

the immunosuppressive medications required to avoid organ rejection.[83] In addition, it has been documented that tumor behavior is often more aggressive in these patients, displaying features such as deeper penetration, infiltrative growth pattern, perineural or lymphatic invasion, and higher risk for recurrence (Figure 1.3).[84,85,86] However, a recent retrospective case-control study of Mohs surgery in transplant patients demonstrated that the individual surgical defects were not significantly larger than those in control subjects. In the same study, there was no statistically significant difference between repair types used in the two groups.[87] Nonetheless, the increased tumor burden in transplant patients over time may result in a greater number of lifetime skin cancer treatments. The consequential accumulation of scars can impact skin laxity within a cosmetic subunit, thereby affecting primary closures, and decrease the size of the available tissue reservoir for flap repairs.

Murine studies suggest that tumor size may be affected in different ways by various immunosuppressant agents. Mice exposed to ultraviolet B light developed significantly larger skin cancers when given cyclosporine or tacrolimus. However, the administration of sirolimus, either alone or in combination with these agents, was associated with an increased number of tumors with a decreased individual tumor size. Similarly, mycophenolate mofetil also correlated with decreased tumor size when added to cyclosporine.[88] Additional studies are needed to determine the relevance of these findings to patient care.

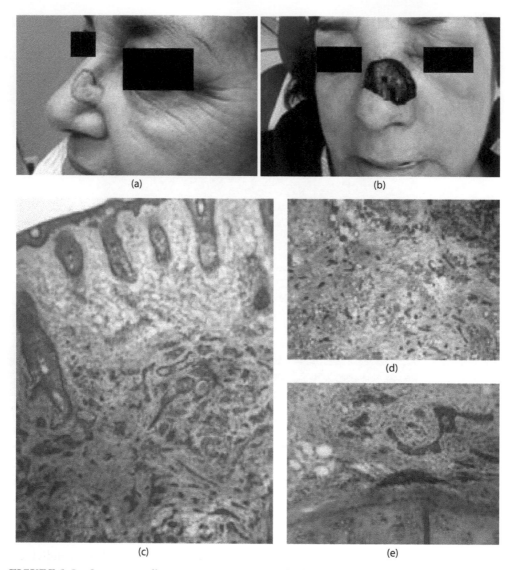

FIGURE 1.3 Squamous cell carcinoma in a patient with a history of liver transplant. (a) Before Mohs surgery. (b) Postoperative defect, demonstrating a through-and-through involvement of the nasal cavity. (c) Sclerosing pattern, (d) deep infiltration between muscle fibers, and (e) perichondral involvement were noted histologically. (c, d) Original magnification, ×40. (e) Original magnification, ×100.

Side effects of immunosuppressive agents may also have an impact on the perioperative course. Most notably, the risk for wound infections is increased due to decreased resistance to pathogens. Certain immunosuppressive medications may also directly have an impact on the wound healing process. In particular, sirolimus has been associated with an increased incidence of surgical complications.[89] When studied retrospectively in dermatological surgery patients, wound dehiscence occurred in 7.7% of sirolimus patients, compared to 0% of controls. This finding was not statistically significant, but it may have been affected by a small sample size.[90]

Neutropenia is another potential adverse effect of some immunosuppressive medications, but it may also occur in patients undergoing cancer chemotherapy. As previously discussed, neutrophils are the first inflammatory cells involved in the wound healing process. Impaired healing has been observed in neutropenic patients, a finding that can be partially reversed by the administration of granulocyte colony-stimulating factor (G-CSF).[91,92] Furthermore, neutropenic patients are at high risk for bacterial infections. Therefore, in situations where neutrophil counts are expected to improve, such as following a round of chemotherapy, consideration should be given to briefly delaying Mohs surgery if the clinical context allows.

Systemic corticosteroids also cause immunosuppression and may impair wound healing, but with a clinical impact that varies depending on chronicity. Thus, acute, high doses of systemic corticosteroids for less than 10 days prior to surgery are unlikely to affect subsequent healing. However, chronic use for more than 30 days is associated with a two- to fivefold increase in the risk for wound healing complications.[93]

Systemic Retinoids

Since nonmelanoma skin cancers are on the rise in young adults,[94] Mohs surgeons may increasingly encounter patients who have been exposed to oral isotretinoin in the perioperative period. Anecdotal reports of scarring and abnormal wound healing following isotretinoin administration have previously been published.[95,96] As a result, traditional teaching has been to avoid cosmetic procedures for 6–12 months following the discontinuation of the medication. Recent evidence, however, contradicts this viewpoint, as resurfacing procedures during isotretinoin therapy did not produce abnormal scarring in two recent studies.[97,98] Furthermore, animal models demonstrate normal characteristics of wound healing despite exposure to this agent.[99,100] Therefore, the current evidence suggests that isotretinoin use is unlikely to increase the risk for wound complications or to result in poorer aesthetic outcomes following Mohs surgery.

More commonly, Mohs surgeons may encounter patients who have been prescribed oral acitretin. In addition to the more common indications, such as psoriasis, this medication is also sometimes used for chemoprevention of squamous cell carcinoma in high-risk patients, such as those with a history of organ transplants. One study demonstrated that acitretin does not significantly impact wound healing following reconstruction or by second intent.[101]

Anticoagulants and Coagulation Disorders

Hemorrhagic complications following Mohs surgery can lead to several sequelae that can adversely affect the final cosmetic result. These include hematoma and seroma formation, wound dehiscence, flap necrosis, graft failure, and infection. It is essential that patients at risk for bleeding be identified preoperatively to minimize risk.

Bleeding diatheses can be divided into acquired and congenital types. In the acquired category, patients most commonly encountered by a Mohs surgeon are those taking prescription or over-the-counter anticoagulants, including herbal supplements. Additional acquired causes include liver failure, uremia, vitamin K deficiency, leukemia, thrombocytopenia (for example, idiopathic thrombocytopenic purpura), and autoimmune coagulopathies. Less often, a patient may have an inherited bleeding disorder.

It is estimated that 25% to 38% of patients presenting for Mohs surgery are on anticoagulant drugs.[102] These medications include aspirin, nonsteroidal anti-inflammatory drugs (NSAIDs), clopidogrel, warfarin, and newer anticoagulants such as dabigatran, apixaban, rivaroxaban, and argatroban. It should be noted that bleeding complications in Mohs surgery are rare, occurring in approximately 0.1% of patients; the majority of patients with this complication are on anticoagulant medications.[103,104]

Given the low risk for hemorrhagic complications in dermatological surgery relative to the potential morbidity and mortality associated with a potential thrombotic event, current recommendations are to continue anticoagulant medications during the perioperative period.[102,105] An exception to these recommendations includes the cessation of aspirin when used for primary prevention of myocardial infarction and stroke and of other NSAIDs when used for pain relief.[106] In addition, patients may be taking one of several herbal preparations that possess an anticoagulant effect. These include ginkgo biloba, vitamin E, feverfew, ginger, ginseng, garlic, fish oil, and saw palmetto (when combined with warfarin). It is recommended that these supplements be stopped in the perioperative period.[106]

Other acquired causes of abnormal bleeding may require additional interventions prior to dermatological surgery, but typically only in the most severe cases. For example, liver failure results in decreased synthesis of several coagulation factors. In severe cases, these can be infused intraoperatively. While most causes of thrombocytopenia do not result in clinically significant bleeding, platelet counts below 20,000/mL may not be sufficient to prevent postoperative hemorrhage. In such cases, platelet infusion may be necessary prior to surgery.

In addition, at least 1% of the population is affected by one of the three most common coagulation disorders: von Willebrand disease, hemophilia A, and hemophilia B. Ideally, identification of these patients would occur through the preoperative history. A multidisciplinary approach in coordination with hematology should be considered, as certain therapies, such as factor replacement, may be available. Meticulous hemostasis, careful selection of reconstructive techniques, and close postoperative follow-up are essential in such cases.[107]

Nutritional Status

It is well documented that malnutrition is associated with delayed wound healing and an increased susceptibility to infection.[108] Therefore, patients with protein malnutrition, such as that resulting from chronic disease, chronic infection, recent hospitalization, or prior gastrointestinal surgery, should be counseled on their risk for slow wound healing. In severe cases, it is appropriate to discuss perioperative protein supplementation.

Zinc has been an ancient health remedy since at least Roman times.[109] More specific to surgery, zinc supplementation was shown over 50 years ago to accelerate healing of granulating wounds.[110] It has also become clear that this element plays a key role in each phase of the wound healing process and possesses anti-inflammatory properties. For example, zinc-deficient rats have delayed reepithelialization and decreased scar strength.[111] However, more recent studies addressing oral supplementation for wounds in human subjects suggest a benefit only for individuals predisposed to low levels of zinc.[112] Thus, it remains unclear whether supplementation has a similar effect on wound healing in those without a preexisting zinc deficiency.

Vitamin C stimulates the immune system, strengthens connective tissue, and promotes wound healing, such that its profound deficiency in the form of scurvy can result in open suppurative wounds, among other well-described features.[113] Studies investigating the potential benefits of vitamin C supplementation on postoperative scarring in healthy individuals have shown conflicting results. Thus, there is insufficient evidence that either supplementation or experimental partial depletion of vitamin C has significant impact on wound healing.[114,115]

Vascular Abnormalities

Adequate circulation is crucial to achieve optimal wound healing. This concept is most pertinent to Mohs and dermatological surgery when used in the treatment of lower extremity wounds. Defects in this area can be difficult to repair by primary closure, due to limited tissue laxity at baseline, and can subsequently be complicated by wound dehiscence. Lower extremity edema compounds this challenge, and chronic venous insufficiency is commonly encountered, with reports of prevalence ranging from less than 1% to 40% in females and from less than 1% to 17% in males.[116] Diminished arterial flow also impairs wound healing and is commonly seen in clinical practice, with prevalence estimated to be as high as 19.8% in men and 16.8% in women, based on ankle-brachial index measurements in one large German cohort.[117] Chronic lymphedema poses similar challenges to the surgeon and is sometimes encountered in patients following radical mastectomy with axillary lymph node dissection or radiation therapy for breast cancer.

Preoperatively, patients with impaired circulation should be identified based on clinical examination (Figure 1.4). Potential complications should be discussed with the patient; these include increased risk of infection, dehiscence, and flap or graft failure, as well as prolonged healing time. Compression devices may be helpful in the postoperative period for patients with chronic venous insufficiency or chronic lymphedema. These and other interventions designed to optimize wound healing in such patients will be covered in greater detail in Chapter 3.

Hypertension

Patients should be instructed to take their antihypertensive medications as prescribed in the pre- and postoperative periods. In our practices, all surgical patients have their blood

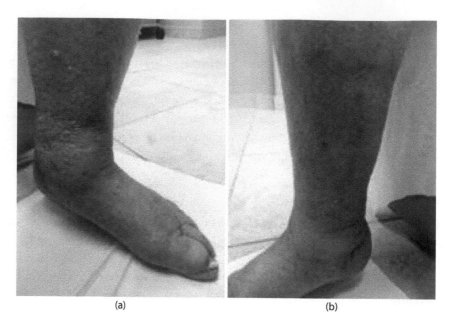

(a)   (b)

FIGURE 1.4   (a, b) Severe stasis changes in a diabetic, hypertensive male patient, including erythema, edema, hemosiderin deposition, early elephantiasis, and lipodermatosclerosis. Surgical intervention carries a very high risk of complications.

pressure checked preoperatively. When performing Mohs surgery, the authors have cutoff values of 180 mm Hg systolic and 100 mm Hg diastolic for an asymptomatic patient.

Although this is somewhat arbitrary, in our experience blood pressures above these values are associated with increased postoperative complications, in particular excessive bleeding. If the preoperative blood pressure cannot be lowered below these levels with simple relaxation maneuvers, surgery is deferred until the hypertension has been appropriately managed.

Prophylactic Antibiotics

Prophylactic antibiotics prior to cutaneous surgery are recommended for patients at high risk for endocarditis or prosthetic joint infection, based on current guidelines that have been summarized.[118] More relevant to the current discussion is whether antibiotic prophylaxis prior to Mohs surgery may result in superior cosmetic outcomes by preventing surgical site infections, which can contribute to wound dehiscence, slow healing, and abnormal scarring.

At baseline, surgical site infections following Mohs surgery are rare, with reported rates generally ranging between less than 1% and 4.25%.[119,120,121] A recent multicenter study of 20,821 Mohs procedures reported an infection rate of 0.39%.[103] Consistent with this low risk, Wright et al. recommended limiting antibiotic prophylaxis to those sites and scenarios that carry higher risk for surgical infection. These include wounds on the lower extremity or in the groin, wedge excisions on the lip or ear, reconstruction using a skin flap on the nose or a skin graft on any site, and presence of extensive inflammatory skin disease.[118]

Antibiotic prophylaxis has also been advocated by some authors for other patients at high risk for surgical site infections, including diabetics, smokers, and those with underlying immunosuppression.[122] However, the decision to prescribe antibiotics should be made on a case-by-case basis. Widespread antibiotic use is unnecessary given the low risk of surgical site infections, the potential for the development of antibiotic resistance, and the risk of morbidity associated with these medications.

CONCLUSIONS

Wound healing is an intricate process that continues to be elucidated. For the sake of convenience, this process is typically subdivided into phases, though the actual progression of cellular and molecular events within a wound is continuous.

Due to its complexity, the wound healing process may be significantly affected by various patient factors, which can then result in alterations in the final surgical outcome. Identifying these factors preoperatively is of the utmost importance to help maximize the aesthetic result.

REFERENCES

1. Donaldson MR, Coldiron BM. Dermatologists perform the majority of cutaneous reconstructions in the Medicare population: Numbers and trends from 2004 to 2009. *J Am Acad Dermatol* 2013;68(5):803–8.
2. Kainoh M, Ikeda Y, Nishio S, Nakadate T. Glycoprotein Ia/IIa-mediated activation-dependent platelet adhesion to collagen. *Thromb Res* 1992;65(2):165–76.
3. Pareti FI, Fujimura Y, Dent JA, Holland LZ, Zimmerman TS, Ruggeri ZM. Isolation and characterization of a collagen binding domain in human von Willebrand factor. *J Biol Chem* 1986;261(32):15310–5.
4. Sixma JJ, Sakariassen KS, Stel HV, et al. Functional domains on von Willebrand factor. Recognition of discrete tryptic fragments by monoclonal antibodies that inhibit interaction of von Willebrand factor with platelets and with collagen. *J Clin Invest* 1984;74(3):736–44.
5. Yakushkin VV, Zyuryaev IT, Khaspekova SG, Sirotkina OV, Ruda MY, Mazurov AV. Glycoprotein IIb-IIIa content and platelet aggregation in healthy volunteers and patients with acute coronary syndrome. *Platelets* 2011;22(4):243–51.
6. Naimushin YA, Mazurov AV. Von Willebrand factor can support platelet aggregation via interaction with activated GPIIb-IIIa and GPIb. *Platelets* 2004;15(7):419–25.
7. Ikeda Y, Murata M, Araki Y, et al. Importance of fibrinogen and platelet membrane glycoprotein IIb/IIIa in shear-induced platelet aggregation. *Thromb Res* 1988;51(2):157–63.
8. Yomo T, Serna DL, Powell LL, et al. Glycoprotein IIb/IIIa receptor inhibitor attenuates platelet aggregation induced by thromboxane A2 during in vitro nonpulsatile ventricular assist circulation. *Artif Organs* 2000;24(5):355–61.
9. Repesh LA, Fitzgerald TJ, Furcht LT. Fibronectin involvement in granulation tissue and wound healing in rabbits. *J Histochem Cytochem* 1982;30(4):351–8.
10. Murphy-Ullrih JE, Mosher DF. Localization of thrombospondin in clots formed in situ. *Blood* 1985;66(5):1098–104.
11. Claesson-Welsh L. Mechanism of action of platelet-derived growth factor. *Int J Biochem Cell Biol* 1996;28(4):373–85.
12. Soma Y, Mizoguchi M, Yamane K, et al. Specific inhibition of human skin fibroblast chemotaxis to platelet-derived growth factor A-chain homodimer by transforming growth factor-β1. *Arch Dermatol Res* 2002;293(12):609–13.
13. Grainger DJ, Wakefield L, Bethell HW, Farndale RW, Metcalfe JC. Release and activation of platelet latent TGF-beta in blood clots during dissolution with plasmin. *Nat Med* 1995;1(9):932–7.

14. Postlethwaite AE, Keski-Oja J, Moses HL, Kang AH. Stimulation of the chemotactic migration of human fibroblasts by transforming growth factor β. *J Exp Med* 1987;165(1):251–6.
15. Pierce GF, Mustoe TA, Lingelbach J, et al. Platelet-derived growth factor and transforming growth factor-β enhance tissue repair activities by unique mechanisms. *J Cell Biol* 1989;109(1):429–40.
16. Malik AR, Lo SK. Vascular endothelial adhesion molecules and tissue inflammation. *Pharmacol Rev* 1996;48(2):213–29.
17. Wagner JG, Roth RA. Neutrophil migration mechanisms, with an emphasis on the pulmonary vasculature. *Pharmacol Rev* 2000;52(3):349–74.
18. Cepinskas G, Noseworthy R, Kvietys PR. Transendothelial neutrophil migration. Role of neutrophil-derived proteases and relationship to transendothelial protein movement. *Circ Res* 1997;81(4):618–26.
19. Deuel TF, Senior RM, Huang JS, Griffin GL. Chemotaxis of monocytes and neutrophils to platelet-derived growth factor. *J Clin Invest* 1982;69(4):1046–9.
20. Bar-Shavit R, Kahn A, Fenton JW 2nd, Wilner GD. Chemotactic response of monocytes to thrombin. *J Cell Biol* 1983;96(1):282–5.
21. Wahl SM, Hunt DA, Wakefield LM, et al. Transforming growth factor type β induces monocyte chemotaxis and growth factor production. *Proc Natl Sci U S A* 1987;84(16):5788–92.
22. Deshmane SL, Kremlev S, Amini S, Sawaya BE. Monocyte chemoattractant protein-1 (MCP-1): An overview. *J Interferon Cytokine Res* 2009;29(6):313–26.
23. Mahdavian Delavary B, van der Veer WM, van Egmond M, Niessen FB, Beelen RH. Macrophages in skin injury and repair. *Immunobiology* 2011;216(7):753–62.
24. Koh TJ, DiPietro LA. Inflammation and wound healing: The role of the macrophage. *Expert Rev Mol Med* 2011;13:e23.
25. Falanga V. Growth factors and wound healing. *J Dermatol Surg Oncol* 1993;19(8):711–4.
26. Mirza R, DiPietro LA, Koh TJ. Selective and specific macrophage ablation is detrimental to wound healing in mice. *Am J Pathol* 2009;175(6):2454–62.
27. Goren I, Allmann N, Yogev N, et al. A transgenic mouse model of inducible macrophage depletion: Effects of diphtheria toxin-driven lysozyme M-specific cell lineage ablation on wound inflammatory, angiogenic, and contractive processes. *Am J Pathol* 2009;175(1):132–47.
28. Plikus MV, Gay DL, Treffeisen E, Wang A, Supapannachart RJ, Cotsarelis G. Epithelial stem cells and implications for wound repair. *Semin Cell Dev Biol* 2012;23(9):946–53.
29. Ito M, Liu Y, Yang Z, et al. Stem cells in the hair follicle bulge contribute to wound repair but not to homeostasis of the epidermis. *Nat Med* 2005;11(12):1351–4.
30. Peplow PV, Chatterjee MP. A review of the influence of growth factors and cytokines in in vitro human keratinocyte migration. *Cytokine* 2013;62(1):1–21.
31. Brauchle M, Angermeyer K, Hübner G, Werner S. Large induction of keratinocyte growth factor expression by serum growth factors and pro-inflammatory cytokines in cultured fibroblasts. *Oncogene* 1994;9(11):3199–204.
32. Safferling K, Sütterlin T, Westphal K, et al. Wound healing revised: A novel reepithelialization mechanism revealed by in vitro and in silico models. *J Cell Biol* 2013;203(4):691–709.
33. Nobes CD, Hall A. Rho, rac and cdc42 GTPases: Regulators of actin structures, cell adhesion and motility. *Biochem Soc Trans* 1995;23(3):456–9.
34. Pilcher BK, Dumin JA, Sudbeck BD, Krane SM, Welgus HG, Parks WC. The activity of collagenase-1 is required for keratinocyte migration on a type I collagen matrix. *J Cell Biol* 1997;137(6):1445–57.
35. Sudbeck BD, Pilcher BK, Welgus HG, Parks WC. Induction and repression of collagenase-1 by keratinocytes is controlled by distinct components of different extracellular matrix compartments. *J Biol Chem* 1997;272(35):22103–10.
36. Puccinelli TJ, Bertics PJ, Masters KS. Regulation of keratinocyte signaling and function via changes in epidermal growth factor presentation. *Acta Biomater* 2010;6(9):3415–25.
37. Sun T, Adra S, Smallwood R, Holcombe M, MacNeil S. Exploring hypotheses of the actions of TGF-β1 in epidermal wound healing using a 3D computational multiscale model of the human epidermis. *PLoS One* 2009;4(12):e8515.
38. Gibbs S, Silva Pinto AN, Murli S, Huber M, Hohl D, Ponec M. Epidermal growth factor and keratinocyte growth factor differentially regulate epidermal migration, growth, and differentiation. *Wound Repair Regen* 2000;8(3):192–203.

39. Beer HD, Gassmann MG, Munz B, et al. Expression and function of keratinocyte growth factor and activin in skin morphogenesis and cutaneous wound repair. *J Investig Dermatol Symp Proc* 2000;5(1):34–9.

40. Tonnesen MG, Feng X, Clark RA. Angiogenesis in wound healing. *J Investig Dermatol Symp Proc* 2000;5(1):40–6.

41. Lawler PR, Lawler J. Molecular basis for the regulation of angiogenesis by thrombospondin-1 and -2. *Cold Spring Harb Perspect Med* 2012;2(5):a006627.

42. Kalebic T, Garbisa S, Glaser B, Liotta LA. Basement membrane collagen: Degradation by migrating endothelial cells. *Science* 1983;221(4607):281–3.

43. Takehara K. Growth regulation of skin fibroblasts. *J Dermatol Sci* 2000;24 Suppl 1:S70–S7.

44. Postlethwaite AE, Keski-Oja J, Moses HL, Kang AH. Stimulation of the chemotactic migration of human fibroblasts by transforming growth factor β. *J Exp Med* 1987;165(1):251–6.

45. Smith AN, Willis E, Chan VT, et al. Mesenchymal stem cells induce dermal fibroblast responses to injury. *Exp Cell Res* 2010;316(1):48–54.

46. Clark RA. Fibronectin matrix deposition and fibronectin receptor expression in healing and normal skin. *J Invest Dermatol* 1990;94 Suppl 6:128S–34S.

47. Glim JE, Niessen FB, Everts V, van Egmond M, Beelen RH. Platelet derived growth factor-CC secreted by M2 macrophages induces alpha-smooth muscle actin expression by dermal and gingival fibroblasts. *Immunobiology* 2013;218(6):924–9.

48. Desmoulière A, Geinoz A, Gabbiani F, Gabbiani G. Transforming growth factor-β 1 induces α-smooth muscle actin expression in granulation tissue myofibroblasts and in quiescent and growing cultured fibroblasts. *J Cell Biol* 1993;122(1):103–11.

49. Fujiwara T, Kubo T, Kanazawa S, et al. Direct contact of fibroblasts with neuronal processes promotes differentiation to myofibroblasts and induces contraction of collagen matrix in vitro. *Wound Repair Regen* 2013;21(4):588–94.

50. Frazier K, Williams S, Kothapalli D, Klapper H, Grotendorst GR. Stimulation of fibroblast cell growth, matrix production, and granulation tissue formation by connective tissue growth factor. *J Invest Dermatol* 1996;107(3):404–11.

51. Igarashi A, Okochi H, Bradham DM, Grotendorst GR. Regulation of connective tissue growth factor gene expression in human skin fibroblasts and during wound repair. *Mol Biol Cell* 1993; 4(6):637–45.

52. Grotendorst GR. Connective tissue growth factor: A mediator of TGF-β action on fibroblasts. *Cytokine Growth Factor Rev* 1997;8(3):171–9.

53. Uitto J, Booth BA, Polak KL. Collagen biosynthesis by human skin fibroblasts. II. Isolation and further characterization of type I and type III procollagens synthesized in culture. *Biochim Biophys Acta* 1980;624(2):545–61.

54. Pickett BP, Burgess LP, Livermore GH, Tzikas TL, Vossoughi J. Wound healing. Tensile strength vs. healing time for wounds closed under tension. *Arch Otolaryngol Head Neck Surg* 1996;122(5):565–8.

55. Morin G, Rand M, Burgess LP, Voussoughi J, Graeber GM. Wound healing: Relationship of wound closing tension to tensile strength in rats. *Laryngoscope* 1989;99(8 Pt 1):783–8.

56. Horstmeyer A, Licht C, Scherr G, Eckes B, Krieg T. Signalling and regulation of collagen I synthesis by ET-1 and TGF-β1. *FEBS J* 2005;272(24):6297–309.

57. Reed MJ, Vernon RB, Abrass IB, Sage EH. TGF-beta 1 induces the expression of type I collagen and SPARC, and enhances contraction of collagen gels, by fibroblasts from young and aged donors. *J Cell Physiol* 1994;158(1):169–79.

58. Namazi MR, Fallahzadeh MK, Schwartz RA. Strategies for prevention of scars: What can we learn from fetal skin? *Int J Dermatol* 2011;50(1):85–93.

59. Ulrich D, Ulrich F, Unglaub F, Piatkowski A, Pallua N. Matrix metalloproteinases and tissue inhibitors of metalloproteinases in patients with different types of scars and keloids. *J Plast Reconstr Aesthet Surg* 2010;63(6):1015–21.

60. Simon F, Bergeron D, Larochelle S, et al. Enhanced secretion of TIMP-1 by human hypertrophic scar keratinocytes could contribute to fibrosis. *Burns* 2012;38(3):421–7.

61. Oliveira GV, Hawkins HK, Chinkes D, et al. Hypertrophic versus non hypertrophic scars compared by immunohistochemistry and laser confocal microscopy: Type I and III collagens. *Int Wound J* 2009;6(6):445–52.

62. Eckes B, Zweers MC, Zhang ZG, et al. Mechanical tension and integrin alpha 2 beta 1 regulate fibroblast functions. *J Investig Dermatol Symp Proc* 2006;11(1):66–72.
63. Rustad KC, Wong VW, Gurtner GC. The role of focal adhesion complexes in fibroblast mechano-transduction during scar formation. *Differentiation* 2013;86(3):87–91.
64. Medina A, Ghaffari A, Kilani RT, Ghahary A. The role of stratifin in fibroblast-keratinocyte interaction. *Mol Cell Biochem* 2007;305(1-2):255–64.
65. Bond JE, Ho TQ, Selim MA, Hunter CL, Bowers EV, Levinson H. Temporal spatial expression and function of non-muscle myosin II isoforms IIA and IIB in scar remodeling. *Lab Invest* 2011;91(4):499–508.
66. Desmouliere A, Chaponnier C, Gabbiani G. Tissue repair, contraction, and the myofibroblast. *Wound Repair Regen* 2005;13(1):7–12.
67. Abe M, Yokoyama Y, Ishikawa O. A possible mechanism of basic fibroblast growth factor-promoted scarless wound healing: The induction of myofibroblast apoptosis. *Eur J Dermatol* 2012;22(1):46–53.
68. Wietecha MS, Cerny WL, DiPietro LA. Mechanisms of vessel regression: Toward an understanding of the resolution of angiogenesis. *Curr Top Microbiol Immunol* 2013;367:3–32.
69. Lan CC, Liu IH, Fang AH, Wen CH, Wu CS. Hyperglycaemic conditions decrease cultured keratinocyte mobility: Implications for impaired wound healing in patients with diabetes. *Br J Dermatol* 2008;159(5):1103–15.
70. Christman AL, Selvin E, Margolis DJ, Lazarus GS, Garza LA. Hemoglobin A1c predicts healing rate in diabetic wounds. *J Invest Dermatol* 2011;131(10):2121–7.
71. Mosely LH, Finseth F, Goody M. Nicotine and its effect on wound healing. *Plast Reconstr Surg* 1978;61(4):570–5.
72. Sørensen LT. Wound healing and infection in surgery: The pathophysiological impact of smoking, smoking cessation, and nicotine replacement therapy: A systematic review. *Ann Surg* 2012;255(6):1069–79.
73. Monfrecola G, Riccio G, Savarese C, Posteraro G, Procaccini EM. The acute effect of smoking on cutaneous microcirculation blood flow in habitual smokers and nonsmokers. *Dermatology* 1998;197(2):115–8.
74. Lawrence WT, Murphy RC, Robson MC, Heggers JP. The detrimental effect of cigarette smoking on flap survival: An experimental study in the rat. *Br J Plast Surg* 1984;37(2):216–9.
75. Møller AM, Villebro N, Pedersen T, Tønnesen H. Effect of preoperative smoking intervention on postoperative complications: A randomised clinical trial. *Lancet* 2002;359(9301):114–7.
76. Ranzer MJ, Chen L, Dipietro LA. Fibroblast function and wound breaking strength is impaired by acute ethanol intoxication. *Alcohol Clin Exp Res* 2011;35(1):83–90.
77. Stephens P, al-Khateeb T, Davies KJ, Shepherd JP, Thomas DW. An investigation of the interaction between alcohol and fibroblasts in wound healing. *Int J Oral Maxillofac Surg* 1996;25(2):161–4.
78. Peltz S. Severe thrombocytopenia secondary to alcohol use. *Postgrad Med* 1991;89(6):75–6,85.
79. Renaud SC, Beswick AD, Fehily AM, Sharp DS, Elwood PC. Alcohol and platelet aggregation: The Caerphilly Prospective Heart Disease Study. *Am J Clin Nutr* 1992;55(5):1012–7.
80. Haut MJ, Cowan DH. The effect of ethanol on hemostatic properties of human blood platelets. *Am J Med* 1974;56(1):22–33.
81. Meade TW, Chakrabarti R, Haines AP, North WR, Stirling Y. Characteristics affecting fibrinolytic activity and plasma fibrinogen concentrations. *Br Med J* 1979;1(6157):153–6.
82. Sierksma A, van der Gaag MS, Kluft C, Hendriks HF. Moderate alcohol consumption reduces plasma C-reactive protein and fibrinogen levels; a randomized, diet-controlled intervention study. *Eur J Clin Nutr* 2002;56(11):1130–6.
83. Zwald FO, Brown M. Skin cancer in solid organ transplant recipients: Advances in therapy and management: Part I. Epidemiology of skin cancer in solid organ transplant recipients. *J Am Acad Dermatol* 2011;65(2):253–61.
84. Lott DG, Manz R, Koch C, Lorenz RR. Aggressive behavior of nonmelanotic skin cancers in solid organ transplant recipients. *Transplantation* 2010;90(6):683–7.
85. Buell JF, Hanaway MJ, Thomas M, Alloway RR, Woodle ES. Skin cancer following transplantation: The Israel Penn International Transplant Tumor Registry experience. *Transplant Proc* 2005;37(2):962–3.

86. Smith KJ, Hamza S, Skelton H. Histologic features in primary cutaneous squamous cell carcinomas in immunocompromised patients focusing on organ transplant patients. *Dermatol Surg* 2004;30(4 Pt 2):634–41.

87. Upjohn E, Bhore R, Taylor RS. Solid organ transplant recipients presenting for Mohs micrographic surgery: A retrospective case-control study. *Dermatol Surg* 2012;38(9):1448–55.

88. Duncan FJ, Wulff BC, Tober KL, et al. Clinically relevant immunosuppressants influence UVB-induced tumor size through effects on inflammation and angiogenesis. *Am J Transplant* 2007;7(12):2693–703.

89. Dean PG, Lund WJ, Larson TS, et al. Wound-healing complications after kidney transplantation: A prospective, randomized comparison of sirolimus and tacrolimus. *Transplantation* 2004;77(10):1555–61.

90. Brewer JD, Otley CC, Christenson LJ, Phillips PK, Roenigk RK, Weaver AL. The effects of sirolimus on wound healing in dermatologic surgery. *Dermatol Surg* 2008;34(2):216–23.

91. Cody DT 2nd, Funk GF, Wagner D, Gidley PW, Graham SM, Hoffman HT. The use of granulocyte colony stimulating factor to promote wound healing in a neutropenic patient after head and neck surgery. *Head Neck* 1999;21(2):172–5.

92. Besner GE, Glick PL, Karp MP, et al. Recombinant human granulocyte colony-stimulating factor promotes wound healing in a patient with congenital neutropenia. *J Pediatr Surg* 1992;27(3):288–90.

93. Wang AS, Armstrong EJ, Armstrong AW. Corticosteroids and wound healing: Clinical considerations in the perioperative period. *Am J Surg* 2013;206(3):410–7.

94. Christenson LJ, Borrowman TA, Vachon CM, et al. Incidence of basal cell and squamous cell carcinomas in a population younger than 40 years. *JAMA* 2005;294(6):681–90.

95. Zachariae H. Delayed wound healing and keloid formation following argon laser treatment or dermabrasion during isotretinoin treatment. *Br J Dermatol* 1988;118(5):703–6.

96. Rubenstein R, Roenigk HH Jr, Stegman SJ, Hanke CW. Atypical keloids after dermabrasion of patients taking isotretinoin. *J Am Acad Dermatol* 1986;15(2 Pt 1):280–5.

97. Bagatin E, dos Santos Guadanhim LR, Yarak S, Kamamoto CS, de Almeida FA. Dermabrasion for acne scars during treatment with oral isotretinoin. *Dermatol Surg* 2010;36(4):483–9.

98. Picosse FR, Yarak S, Cabral NC, Bagatin E. Early chemabrasion for acne scars after treatment with oral isotretinoin. *Dermatol Surg* 2012;38(9):1521–6.

99. Larson DL, Flugstad NA, O'Connor E, Kluesner KA, Plaza JA. Does systemic isotretinoin inhibit healing in a porcine wound model? *Aesthet Surg J* 2012;32(8): 989–98.

100. Moy RL, Moy LS, Bennett RG, Zitelli JA, Uitto J. Systemic isotretinoin: Effects on dermal wound healing in a rabbit ear model in vivo. *J Dermatol Surg Oncol* 1990;16(12):1142–6.

101. Tan SR, Tope WD. Effect of acitretin on wound healing in organ transplant recipients. *Dermatol Surg* 2004;30(4 Pt 2):667–73.

102. Bordeaux JS, Martires KJ, Goldberg D, Pattee SF, Fu P, Maloney ME. Prospective evaluation of dermatologic surgery complications including patients on multiple antiplatelet and anticoagulant medications. *J Am Acad Dermatol* 2011;65(3):576–83.

103. Alam M, Ibrahim O, Nodzenski M, et al. Adverse events associated with Mohs micrographic surgery: Multicenter prospective cohort study of 20,821 cases at 23 centers. *JAMA Dermatol* 2013;149(12):1378–85.

104. Cook-Norris RH, Michaels JD, Weaver AL, et al. Complications of cutaneous surgery in patients taking clopidogrel-containing anticoagulation. *J Am Acad Dermatol* 2011;65(3):584–91.

105. Otley CC. Continuation of medically necessary aspirin and warfarin during cutaneous surgery. *Mayo Clin Proc* 2003;78(11):1392–6.

106. Bunick CG, Aasi SZ. Hemorrhagic complications in dermatologic surgery. *Dermatol Ther* 2011;24(6):537–50.

107. Peterson SR, Joseph AK. Inherited bleeding disorders in dermatologic surgery. *Dermatol Surg* 2001;27(10):885–9.

108. Thompson WD, Ravdin IS, Frank IL. Effect of hypoproteinemia on wound disruption. *Arch Surg* 1938;36:500–8.

109. Giachi G, Pallecchi P, Romualdi A, et al. Ingredients of a 2,000-y-old medicine revealed by chemical, mineralogical, and botanical investigations. *Proc Natl Acad Sci U S A* 2013;110(4):1193–6.

110. Pories WJ, Henzel JH, Rob CG, Strain WH. Acceleration of wound healing in man with zinc sulphate given by mouth. *Lancet* 1967;1(7482):121–4.
111. Schwartz JR, Marsh RG, Draelos ZD. Zinc and skin health: Overview of physiology and pharmacology. *Dermatol Surg* 2005;31(7 Pt 2):837–47.
112. Wilkinson EA. Oral zinc for arterial and venous leg ulcers. *Cochrane Database Syst Rev* 2012;8:CD001273.
113. Crandon, JH, Lund CC, Dil DB. Experimental human scurvy. *N Engl J Med* 1940;223:353–69.
114. Crandon JH, Landau B, Mikal S, Balmanno J, Jefferson M, Mahoney N. Ascorbic acid economy in surgical patients as indicated by blood ascorbic acid levels. *N Engl J Med* 1958;258(3):105–13.
115. Vaxman F, Olender S, Lambert A, et al. Effect of pantothenic acid and ascorbic acid supplementation on human skin wound healing process. A double-blind, prospective and randomized trial. *Eur Surg Res* 1995;27:158–66.
116. Beebe-Dimmer JL, Pfeifer JR, Engle JS, Schottenfeld D. The epidemiology of chronic venous insufficiency and varicose veins. *Ann Epidemiol* 2005;15(3):175–84.
117. Diehm C, Schuster A, Allenberg JR, et al. High prevalence of peripheral arterial disease and comorbidity in 6880 primary care patients: Cross-sectional study. *Atherosclerosis* 2004;172(1):95–105.
118. Wright TI, Baddour LM, Berbari EF, et al. Antibiotic prophylaxis in dermatologic surgery: Advisory statement 2008. *J Am Acad Dermatol* 2008;59(3):464–73.
119. Dixon AJ, Dixon MP, Askew DA, Wilkinson D. Prospective study of wound infections in dermatologic surgery in the absence of prophylactic antibiotics. *Dermatol Surg* 2006;32(6):819–26.
120. Maragh SL, Brown MD. Prospective evaluation of surgical site infection rate among patients with Mohs micrographic surgery without the use of prophylactic antibiotics. *J Am Acad Dermatol* 2008;59(2):275–8.
121. Rogers HD, Desciak EB, Marcus RP, Wang S, MacKay-Wiggan J, Eliezri YD. Prospective study of wound infections in Mohs micrographic surgery using clean surgical technique in the absence of prophylactic antibiotics. *J Am Acad Dermatol* 2010;63(5):842–51.
122. Rossi AM, Mariwalla K. Prophylactic and empiric use of antibiotics in dermatologic surgery: A review of the literature and practical considerations. *Dermatol Surg* 2012;38(12):1898–921.

Chapter 2

Intraoperative Surgical Techniques and Pearls

Laura Kline and Brett Coldiron

INTRODUCTION

Once surgical planning and patient preparation have been accomplished, attention must be turned proper surgical and perioperative techniques that aim to optimize wound healing and minimize surgical complications. While surgeons differ in their choice of specific reconstructive techniques to employ in a given scenario, certain principles can be used as guidelines to maximize aesthetic results. This chapter aims to illustrate the intraoperative techniques that improve outcomes for the patient and the surgeon, and to demonstrate that a simpler approach is often most suitable.

PREOPERATIVE PERIOD

In the surgical suite, the surgical team can take a number of measures to reduce patient anxiety and to set the stage for a successful outcome. From the patient perspective, the complexity of Mohs micrographic surgery can seem overwhelming. Taking the time to educate patients helps alleviate anxiety and manage expectations. Prior to surgery, informative brochures outlining the Mohs procedure and providing details of the clinical practice can be given or sent to patients. These serve as invaluable resources to patients. Simply knowing what to expect alleviates a great deal of concern. Research suggests that preoperative information may reduce anxiety, cortisol levels, and postoperative pain while hastening recovery and increasing patient satisfaction.[1]

Occasionally, patients continue to harbor uncontrolled anxiety. Anxiolytics such as lorazepam, or haloperidol for patients over the age of 65, can further diminish anxiety and perception of pain, contributing to a positive patient experience. Anxiolytics can also help manage elevated blood pressure related to anxiety and diminish the risk of complications related to excessive bleeding. Judicious use of distraction in the form of conversation or music can further promote a positive patient experience. In fact, research has demonstrated that patient-preferred music can help diminish the perception of pain and reduce anxiety during surgical procedures, including Mohs surgery.[2,3]

Taking the time to get to know patients, develop rapport, and recognize particular personality types can greatly enhance the surgical experience. Patients labeled as "difficult" often have personality disorders. The ability to recognize these and to deal with them appropriately rather than defensively can circumvent potential complications. Avoidance of an adversarial relationship is critical.

Other factors contributing to a smooth surgical experience include appropriate lighting, photographs, and instruments. Proper overhead lighting is essential for accurate preoperative tumor delineation. Furthermore, the use of special lighting, such as a Wood's lamp, can help to more accurately distinguish the borders of certain tumors, including maligna lentigo melanoma. Appropriate magnification and gentle stretching of the skin can be of further benefit in delineating the extent of infiltration by nonmelanoma skin cancer. The use of pre-, intra-, and postoperative photographs is also an invaluable resource. Photographs can aid in revealing preexisting facial asymmetries, can serve as objective evidence of postoperative improvement, and can be used to improve accuracy of surgical maps. In addition, photographs can provide an objective record of the surgical procedure should further documentation be required by third parties, such as insurance companies. Finally, having appropriate instruments that have been properly maintained and are easily accessible is also crucial to optimizing outcome and efficiency. Failure to do so can result in unnecessary interruptions to the surgical procedure, which is unsatisfying to both the patient and the surgeon.

INTRAOPERATIVE TECHNIQUES

Anesthesia

Perhaps the most significant source of patient anxiety on the day of surgery is fear of needles and pain. When a patient recollects the surgical experience, the amount of pain experienced during anesthetic injection is likely second in importance only to the appearance of the scar. Delivering the anesthetic in a sensitive manner, while taking advantage of a few techniques to make it less painful, promotes a positive patient experience and can even influence a surgeon's reputation. Techniques that can significantly decrease the sensation of pain include using small-caliber needles (27-gauge or finer), small syringes, slow injection perpendicular to the skin surface, and shaking or pinching the surrounding skin.[4] Minimizing the number of injections, injecting through previously anesthetized skin, and maintaining the solution at room temperature are of added benefit. In our experience, buffering the anesthetic with bicarbonate solution to diminish the pain is not necessary if the above principles are followed.

When possible, regional nerve blocks can also help reduce the discomfort of anesthetic infiltration. Blockage of the infraorbital, supratrochlear, supraorbital, and mental nerves is ideal for anesthetizing particularly sensitive areas, such as the nose and lips; anesthetizing large areas; and reducing the dose of anesthetic (Figure 2.1). In our practice, infraorbital nerve blocks with an intraoral approach are used routinely when operating on the nose. Once the block has taken effect, a small amount of anesthetic with epinephrine can be injected into the surgical site to help with hemostasis. When properly performed, discomfort is significantly decreased.

Soft Tissue Handling

Appropriate technique in handling soft tissues during cutaneous surgery is critical to optimizing wound healing and aesthetic outcome. Appropriate instruments, judicious use of electrosurgical hemostasis, and conservative undermining minimize trauma to the skin and

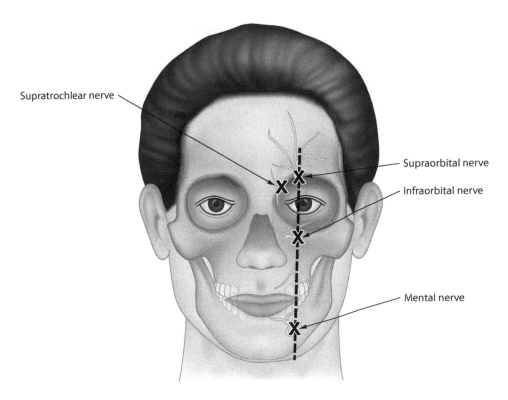

FIGURE 2.1 Landmarks for performing regional nerve blocks on the face: the locations for blocks of the supraorbital, infraorbital, and mental nerves are along one alignment.

subcutaneous tissues. When approximating wound edges or undermining soft tissues, great care must be taken to avoid crush injury to skin edges. Skin hooks can be used as an alternative to forceps; they allow soft tissue to be handled in a significantly less traumatic manner. Like forceps, they can be used to evert wound edges during closure, approximate tissue to assess for adequate undermining, and mobilize flaps over primary defects. Furthermore, skin hooks are superior to forceps in reflecting wound edges to obtain uniform undermining and for attempting to visualize sites of hemorrhage. Selection of instruments proportional to both wound and needle size allows for easier closure of incisions. For example, a small Castroviejo needle driver facilitates appropriate wrist pronation and easily accommodates small needles. These features make it ideal for precise suture placement and handling of delicate facial soft tissues. The use of needle holders with the capability to cut suture also maximizes efficiency.

Soft tissue dissection is essential for closing a wound without tension. Redraping of skin is limited by the tethering effect of fascial connections to underlying bony structures. Undermining the skin releases these attachments and allows the skin to slide freely over the underlying soft tissues. Dissection should be performed uniformly, in a plane that closely matches the depth of the primary defect. Awareness of important underlying anatomic structures also helps guide the path of undermining and is essential to avoiding transection of important nerves and vessels. While some locations, such as the subgaleal plane of the scalp, allow for blunt dissection, sharp dissection with direct visualization is generally preferred.

Sharp dissection allows for greater precision, resulting in less soft tissue trauma. When executed appropriately, undermining allows wound edges to be easily approximated, contributing to a less conspicuous scar. In contrast, inadequate undermining causes increased tissue stretch as wound edges are apposed, compromising the skin's microcirculation and elevating the risk of skin necrosis.[5] However, it is important to recognize that wide undermining does not continue to further decrease closure tension but may instead increase the risk for hematoma formation, compromise blood flow, and result in nerve damage.[6] Undermining is necessary only to the degree that it relieves tension on the wound margins.

If appropriate undermining has not released tension sufficiently, techniques that take advantage of cutaneous mechanical creep can be utilized. These techniques include use of pulley sutures or instruments such as towel clamps to elicit further extensibility of the skin. A towel clamp can be inserted on each side of the wound to more closely approximate wound edges while suturing. However, this technique may leave small puncture scars. The pulley suture is a modification of the vertical mattress suture technique, whereby instead of being tied at the end of execution, the suture is first looped back through the external loop on the contralateral side and then pulled across.[7] Like towel clamps, this stitch can be used to reduce tension while suturing the wound.

Another suturing technique to address elliptical wounds under tension—the subcutaneous corset plication—has also been described. A running suture is placed within the adipose and fascia in the wound base below the undermining plane. The suture is then pulled and tied, reducing the size of the defect.[8] On the scalp, incisions of the galea can help address the limited mobility of the skin in this location.

Hemostasis

Prior to wound closure, meticulous hemostasis should be achieved. Postoperative bleeding significantly increases the risk of necrosis and infection. Furthermore, it is a source of great discomfort and distress for the patient.

Electrosurgery is often used to achieve hemostasis in dermatological surgery. The various modalities include electrodesiccation, electrofulguration, electrocoagulation, electrosection, and electrocautery. Electrocoagulation is a biterminal, monopolar modality with a damped waveform characterized by low-voltage and high-amperage current.[9] Soft tissue provides the necessary resistance to convert electrical energy to heat, resulting in tissue desiccation and protein denaturation.[10] While these properties make it ideal for coagulating small vessels in cutaneous surgery, liberal use creates char, resulting in tissue necrosis, prolongation of wound healing, and increased risk for surgical site infection. Electrocoagulation is performed most effectively in a dry surgical field, since blood dissipates the current from the treatment electrode.[11] Measures such as maintaining a dry surgical field, using the lowest effective power setting and pinpoint-only cautery, and utilizing biterminal forceps facilitate precise, efficient hemostasis while minimizing unintended tissue damage. Biterminal units are safer for patients with implanted electrical devices and can also help avoid electrosurgery-induced dental pain related to metal dental restoration.[12] Electrocoagulation is most effective for actively bleeding vessels <1 mm in diameter and should be carried out meticulously in the wound base. However, skin edges should be spared electrosurgery, since bleeding from the superficial dermal plexus usually resolves with wound closure. For larger vessels, hemostasis may be more successfully achieved with suture ligation. With this method, the complications associated with excessive electrocoagulation are avoided and the risk for delayed bleeding is diminished.

In the authors' experience, short-term application of gentle manual pressure over the surgical site prior to electrocoagulation can make hemostasis much easier to achieve, particularly in patients unable to discontinue anticoagulants. In addition, if the thought of placing a drain in the surgical wound arises, it is likely prudent to perform the procedure to avoid hematoma or seroma formation. A simple Penrose drain fashioned from surgical tubing is sufficient. Hemostasis can often become more complex than anticipated, especially in patients on anti-coagulants. Additional techniques for dealing with bleeding will be presented in Chapter 4.

Reconstructive Planning

Once the tumor has been removed, attention can be turned to reconstructive options. Cosmetic and functional issues must be considered with each wound before a decision is made to allow second intent healing or to cover the wound with a graft or flap. If the risk of tumor recurrence is high, second intent healing or split-thickness skin grafting should be considered, so that any recurrence may be easily detected. Flaps, on the other hand, may conceal a recurrence and delay detection. If tumor recurrence is unlikely and second intent healing is not appropriate, surgical repair can be performed by linear closure, a flap, or a skin graft. In general, the simplest approach often yields the most favorable cosmetic outcome, as well as fewer complications.

The primary objectives should be first preserving proper function, then re-creation of normal anatomy while leaving the least conspicuous scar. Successful design of surgical repairs requires a thorough understanding of skin tension lines, cosmetic subunits, free margins, tissue biomechanics, and soft tissue anatomy. Incisions designed within or parallel to skin tension lines minimize tension on the wound, heal faster, and leave less noticeable scars (Figure 2.2).[13] Repair of defects on the forehead is the most notable exception to this principle, as vertical orientation of the incision may offer a more favorable appearance and helps avoid distortion of the eyebrows.

Cosmetic Subunits   Perhaps the most important factor to consider when designing a surgical repair is the neighboring cosmetic unit junctions (Figure 2.3). Structures within a particular cosmetic unit share similar skin color and texture, pore size, elasticity, thickness, and presence or absence of hair. The human eye recognizes various facial features within the context of these cosmetic units. Therefore, scars placed within the junctions of these units help maintain natural contour and symmetry, in contrast to those within a subunit or those that cross over a unit junction. When the incision approaches a cosmetic subunit junction or a free margin, an M-plasty can be used to shorten the incision and to prevent unwanted encroachment and subsequent distortion.[13] Complex surgical defects that span more than

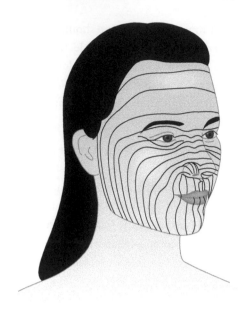

FIGURE 2.2   Relaxed skin tension lines.

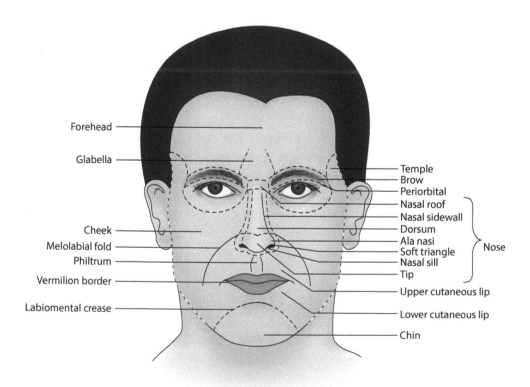

FIGURE 2.3   Cosmetic units and landmarks of the face.

one subunit may require a combination of repairs to keep scars camouflaged within subunit junctions. Adhering to this fundamental principle often means using larger tissue flaps or resecting extra tissue so that suture lines can be placed within a boundary, thus avoiding disruption of the subunit. Counterintuitively, enlarging a surgical defect so as to extend it to its corresponding subunit border, or enlarging the defect so that it occupies the entire cosmetic subunit, can ultimately yield a superior aesthetic result.

Free Margins   An additional principle of importance in surgical reconstruction is the prevention of distortion of free margins. On the face, free margins occur on the eyelid, lip, nasal ala, and nasal tip. The free margins of these structures are more vulnerable to distortion from tension created by surgical movement of tissue. Any disruption of these natural contours not only is aesthetically distracting but also can have negative functional consequences. As discussed in the next chapter, tension vectors directed perpendicular rather than parallel to free margins helps prevent distortion of these structures. Eyebrows should also be given the same consideration as free margins, since they are vulnerable to distortion and asymmetry when placed under tension. Although the skin tension lines are directed horizontally, vertically oriented incisions help avoid unilateral brow elevation. The eyebrow can tolerate up to 5 mm of elevation before the risk of permanent deformity is significant.[13]

Prior to surgical reconstruction, methodical planning should guide selection of the appropriate repair. With the patient in an upright position, skinfolds, relaxed skin tension lines, cosmetic subunits, and free margins should be marked with a surgical pen. These landmarks should be outlined prior to distortion by local anesthetic. Even repairs that appear straightforward should be planned in this manner, ensuring that the aforementioned principles are not violated.

Wound Repair Techniques and Pearls

Second Intent Healing   Although the dermatological surgeon may have a variety of advanced surgical repairs from which to choose, the potential benefit of healing by second intent should be considered. In fact, in appropriately selected wounds, healing by second intent can result in a smaller, more aesthetically pleasing surgical scar.[14] Second intent healing offers a number of important advantages over surgical repair. Granulation allows observation of the wound bed for recurrence of particularly aggressive tumors. For patients unable to endure complex medical procedures, this approach reduces intraoperative time. Wound management is simplified and often less painful. In an era of emphasis on cost containment, second intent healing also decreases the expense of procedures. In addition, complications such as bleeding and infection are rare, while the risk for hematoma, seroma, flap necrosis, or graft loss is avoided entirely. However, patients must be advised that healing will take longer, and they must be counseled on appropriate wound care.

The location of the surgical defect is the most important factor in determining whether healing by second intent will produce an acceptable aesthetic outcome. Areas of concavity on the nose, eye, ear, and temple are known to have favorable outcomes with healing by second intent[15] (Figure 2.4). There is also evidence that flat areas of the forehead, antihelix, eyelid, nose, lip, and cheek heal acceptably by second intent.[16] Small, partial thickness defects are

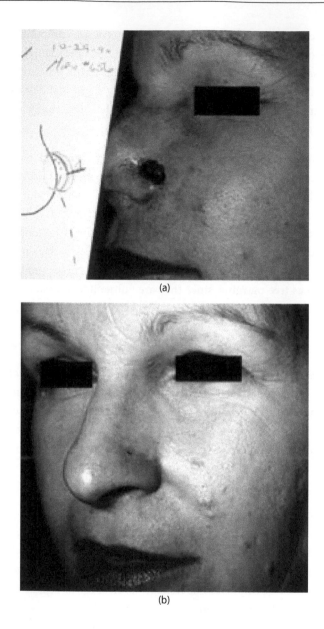

FIGURE 2.4   Healing by second intent can yield superior cosmetic results in concave areas of the nose, eye, ear, and temple. (a) Mohs defect. (b) Appearance after 2 months of healing by second intent, without distortion of the nose or cheek.

especially ideal for healing in this manner. Convex areas of the nose, cheek, chin, and helix predictably heal less favorably by second intent.[17] Furthermore, caution is advised when considering this approach in locations with neighboring free margins, to avoid distortion and functional impairment of the eyelid, lip, or ala.

Layered Closure   If surgical reconstruction is determined to be most beneficial, the next step is careful selection of the appropriate repair. The first consideration on the reconstructive ladder is layered closure. Primary closure is the most common type of reconstruction following Mohs surgery, with approximately half of surgical defects repaired in this manner.[18] It is worth repeating that the simplest approach often confers significant advantage on both the patient and the reconstructive surgeon.

If properly executed, primary closure can result in excellent cosmesis and help avoid complications associated with more complex repairs. Although flaps certainly have their own set of advantages, the geometric angles they require often result in irregularly placed scars that occur perpendicular to the relaxed skin tension lines and natural lines of demarcation. Furthermore, trapdoor deformity is not uncommon with these repairs. With appropriate undermining and adequate removal of dog-ears, even large defects may be repaired with primary closure.[19]

A number of intraoperative techniques can help achieve superior outcomes in primary repairs. Before closure, the surgical defect should be elongated in a fusiform shape, with at least a 3:1 length:width ratio. Wound edges are de-beveled to facilitate wound eversion. Incisions should be executed smoothly, so as not to leave ragged, uneven edges, and should extend to subcutaneous tissue on the first pass. Additionally, incising the inferior aspect before the superior aspect keeps blood from running down and obscuring the surgical field.

An important modification of the primary closure technique addresses the often unnatural appearance of straight-line scars on the face. This is especially true for large incisions that unavoidably cross cosmetic subunits. In such cases, closure should be designed to zigzag across subunit junctions, since the eye does not easily perceive broken lines (Figure 2.5).

Dog-ears should be removed only as needed, not automatically. However, when excision of a dog-ear is required, it should be performed with the intent to remove the redundancy in its entirety. A longer yet smoother scar has a much more favorable appearance than a

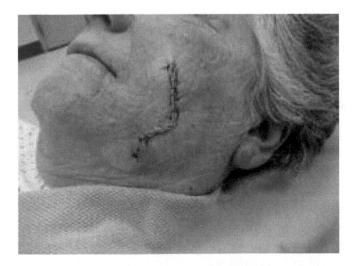

FIGURE 2.5 Changing the direction of the incision when it crosses the jawline allows for a less noticeable scar.

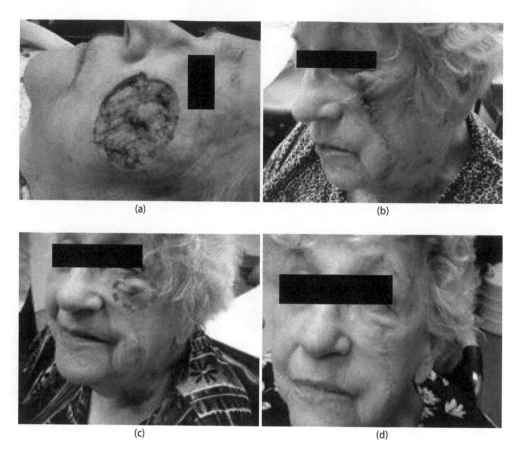

FIGURE 2.6   (a) Defect immediately after Mohs surgery. (b) Appearance at suture removal. The repair is designed so that the tension is perpendicular to the free margin of the eyelid, with redundant tissue remaining superiorly. (c) Appearance at 1 month, with the dog-ear still present. (d) Appearance at 2 months. Note the almost complete disappearance of the dog-ear and absence of distortion of the eyelid.

shorter, puckered scar. In certain anatomic locations, such as the upper extremity and even the infraorbital cheek, dog-ears will settle without requiring excision (Figure 2.6). Beneath the eye, the redundant tissue will help push the eyelid up, lending support to the free margin as the scar contracts. However, in areas of relative skin laxity, such as the lower cheek, dog-ears have a tendency to persist, so they should be removed at the time of closure.

Once appropriate undermining has been performed and hemostasis has been obtained, closure may proceed. Pulling subcutaneous tissue along with dermal sutures is not necessary and results in the need to place more sutures than would otherwise be necessary. Since sutures incite a foreign body inflammatory reaction that can interfere with wound healing and increase the risk of infection, they should be used sparingly. Instead, plication of the subcutaneous fascial tissue with two or three buried absorbable sutures effectively closes the dead space, removes tension from the wound edges, and allows for use of fewer buried sutures (Figure 2.7). These sutures are placed so as to pull subcutaneous tissue together, which in turn approximates tissue edges and relieves tension at the surface.

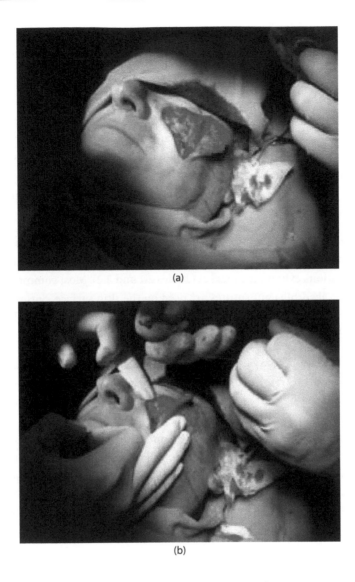

(a)

(b)

FIGURE 2.7   (a) and (b) Plication of fascia closes dead space, relieves tension on the wound, and avoids placement of buried sutures along skin edges.

Suturing Techniques   The surgical incision is now ready for epidermal closure. Proper approximation and eversion of the wound margins is essential to achieving optimal cosmetic outcome. Eversion corrects for the contraction that occurs during the remodeling phase of wound healing. This phenomenon can produce a depressed scar if wound edges are flat at the time of closure. Simple running sutures are often used to close the surface of the skin, and though this technique is effective in rapid wound closure, it may not offer maximal eversion of the wound margins. In the authors' opinion, skin edges cannot be over-everted.

Running horizontal mattress sutures helps maximize eversion and prevent an inverted, depressed scar. This method works particularly well with primary closures. Furthermore, this technique evenly distributes tension across the wound, preventing suture "track marks."

Placing the sutures without undue tension prevents necrosis of skin edges.[20] Although this method of wound closure may not be appropriate for tenuous flaps with narrow pedicles, most primary closures and larger flaps can be closed in this manner.

Placement of running horizontal mattress sutures begins with a simple interrupted suture at the apex of the wound. The needle is then reinserted on the same side as the last exit point, a few millimeters distal to the first suture placement, and exits directly across the wound on the opposite side. Once again, the needle reenters the epidermis a few millimeters distal to the last needle exit and reemerges on the contralateral side. The suture can be periodically tied off to make suture removal easier and ensure even tension across the wound.[20]

Selection of the appropriate suture material and its proper handling are essential for optimized cosmetic outcome. Numerous absorbable and nonabsorbable suture materials in various configurations exist on the market (Tables 2.1 and 2.2). Most commonly, nylon, polypropylene, or fast-absorbing gut sutures are used on the skin surface. Suture material of the smallest caliber minimizes the visibility of the scar and should be used as long as it allows adequate wound approximation.

A needle holder of appropriate size for the needle and the task at hand allows for more precise placement of sutures. The needle is clamped at the body, not at the shank or near the tip, to avoid damage to these more delicate parts of the needle. It also should not be grasped too tightly with the needle driver, to avoid breaking ("springing") the instrument; one "click" of the clamp is usually sufficient. In addition, grasping the suture material with instruments weakens the integrity of the suture and increases the risk of wound dehiscence. Holding the needle driver in the palm allows for maximal wrist pronation and facilitates ease of suture placement. Since the most common needles used in dermatological surgery are curved and have an arc of one-fourth to one-half of a circle, the needle should be guided along this arc rather than forced in a different direction, which can result in needle bending or breaking.

TABLE 2.1   Absorbable Sutures Commonly Used in Dermatological Surgery

Suture Type/ Composition	Configuration	Characteristic Uses in Dermatological Surgery
Plain gut	Monofilament	Skin grafts, mucosal surfaces; rarely used today
Chromic gut	Monofilament	Skin grafts, mucosal surfaces
Fast-absorbing gut	Monofilament	Skin grafts, mucosal surfaces
Polyglycolic acid	Braided multifilament	Subcutaneous tissue approximation, blood vessel ligation
Polyglactin 910	Braided multifilament	Subcutaneous tissue approximation, blood vessel ligation
Polydioxanone	Monofilament	Subcutaneous tissue approximation in high-tension areas
Poliglecaprone 25	Monofilament	Subcutaneous tissue approximation with minimal tissue reactivity

TABLE 2.2   Nonabsorbable Sutures Commonly Used in Dermatological Surgery

Suture Type/ Composition	Configuration	Characteristic Uses in Dermatological Surgery
Nylon	Monofilament or braided multifilament	Used for the majority of surface closures; monofilament associated with reduced risk of infection
Silk	Braided multifilament	Mucosal and intertriginous surfaces
Polypropylene	Monofilament	Subcuticular closures
Polyester	Braided multifilament	Mucosal surfaces

Sutures should be spaced evenly and placed at the same tissue depth to avoid uneven closure. During knot tying, the surgeon's hands and suturing instruments should be kept close to the surgical site. This is much more efficient than chasing large loops of suture material across the surgical field. Also, very tight knots can lead to tissue strangulation. To avoid this complication, only low to moderate tension is placed on the suture ends while tying the first and second knots of a square knot, with only the third knot tied tightly and securely.

Flaps and Grafts   When primary closure is not possible, the next consideration is often a local skin flap or a graft. Cosmetic subunits share similar skin texture, thickness, elasticity, redundancy, and presence or absence of appendageal structures. Therefore, care should be taken to match these tissue characteristics as closely as possible for the best aesthetic outcome. In addition, whenever possible, flaps should be designed to move along cosmetic unit junctures or within relaxed skin tension lines. This is especially true for advancement and rotation flaps, which can be considered elaborate dog-ear repairs or movements of Burow's triangles.

Although a variety of flaps may be used for any particular defect, most of the time the location and size of the defect are the most significant factors in flap selection. While a complete recount of the specific flap designs for every location is beyond the scope of this chapter, the following examples will illustrate the concepts in the previous paragraph.

On the cheek, when the size and location of the defect necessitates closure by means of a local flap, rotation flaps often offer cosmesis superior to that which is possible with transposition flaps. Incisions from transposition flaps often do not conform entirely to relaxed skin tension lines or cosmetic subunit junctions, making the resulting scar more obvious.[21] On the other hand, rotation or advancement flaps on the mid-cheek can often be designed in such a way that the incisions are concealed within the nasolabial fold, the junction of the subunits of the eyelid and infraorbital cheek, or relaxed skin tension lines (Figure 2.8). For defects requiring flap closure on the preauricular cheek, advancement flaps designed to take advantage of the laxity inferior to the defect result in incisions hidden within hair-bearing regions and auricular creases (Figure 2.9).

While primary closure may be performed for most small defects on the chin, for larger defects, rotation flaps or bilateral advancement flaps may be partially concealed in the mental

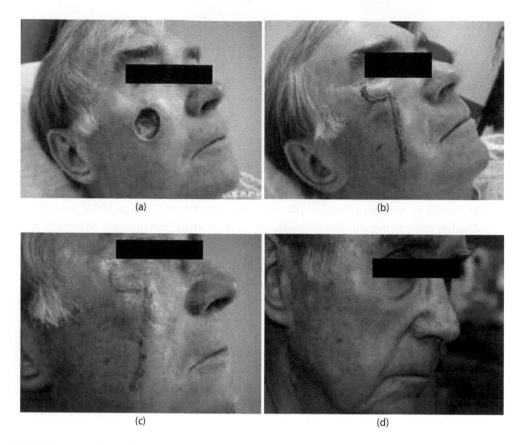

FIGURE 2.8 (a) Mid-cheek defect immediately after Mohs surgery. (b) Incisions placed parallel to relaxed skin tension lines and along cosmetic unit junctions. (c) Appearance at suture removal. (d) Scar camouflaged within the relaxed skin tension lines and along the cosmetic unit junctions of the eyelid and cheek.

crease and marionette lines. Similarly, for large defects of the upper forehead, rotation and advancement flaps can be designed so that incisions are hidden almost entirely within the hair or the hairline (Figure 2.10).

The complex topography of the ear presents unique challenges in surgical reconstruction. For defects on the helical rim, wedge resections or skin grafts have often been used. When wedge excision is executed well, the cosmetic outcome is acceptable. The disadvantages are that this can be a technically difficult repair to perform, particularly for novice surgeons, and that the re-created ear is smaller. With skin grafts, the final appearance often is patch-like and necessitates the creation of a second wound for skin donation. A simpler approach for helical rim defects that are 1.5 cm long or less with intact cartilage and perichondrium is a transposition flap. The tissue is recruited from the postauricular area, creating a secondary defect that can be concealed in the retroauricular sulcus. This defect can often be repaired without buried sutures. The flap is sutured in place, with care taken not to excise dog-ears near the pivot point of the pedicle, which compromises flap vascularity; often these dog-ears improve significantly with time (Figure 2.11).

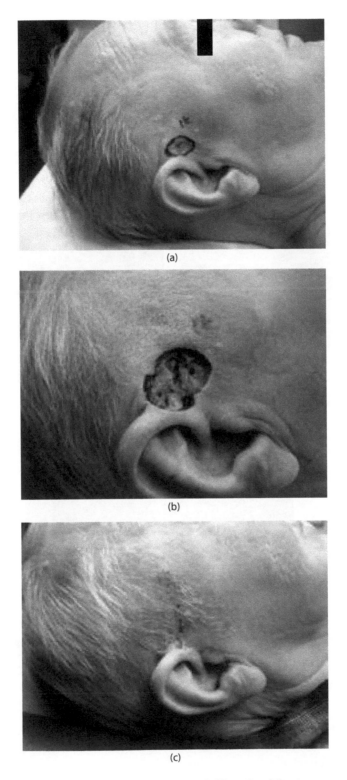

FIGURE 2.9   (a) Preauricular tumor prior to removal. (b) Defect following removal by Mohs surgery. (c) Repair designed to take advantage of the tissue reservoir inferiorly, allowing concealment of the scar within the sideburn and preauricular crease.

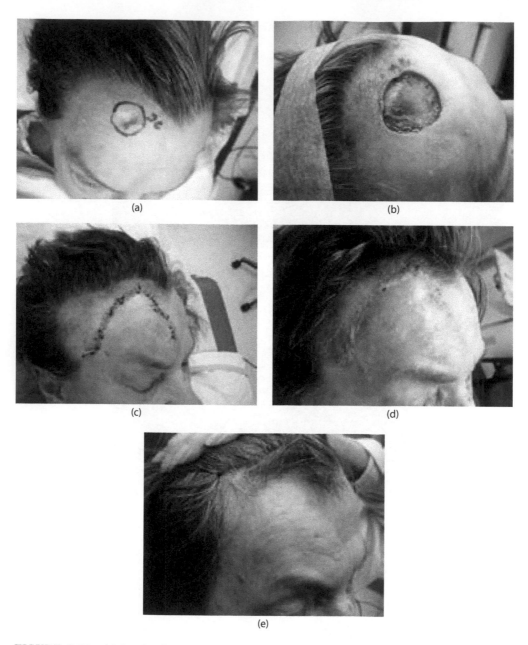

FIGURE 2.10   (a) Basal cell carcinoma of the forehead. (b) Large defect following Mohs surgery. (c) Large rotation flap with the incision mostly concealed along the hairline. (d) Appearance at suture removal. (e) Excellent cosmetic outcome at 2-month follow-up.

Once again, undermining the flap no more than necessary, using plication sutures to relieve tension on wound edges, and minimizing the number of buried sutures helps avoid unwanted complications in flap repairs.

Full-thickness skin grafts can be used on almost any surgical defect with an adequate vascular supply. In addition to matching tissue characteristics, as described in the first paragraph of this section, several other considerations must be taken into account when harvesting and

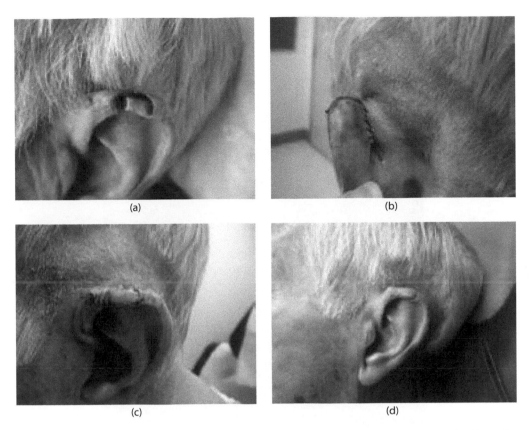

(a)   (b)

(c)   (d)

FIGURE 2.11   (a) Partial-thickness Mohs defect of the helical rim. (b) Transposition flap from the posterior helix. No buried sutures were placed. (c) Standing cone at the base of the flap pedicle usually resolves. (d) Appearance at suture removal. The standing cone has partially resolved.

securing skin grafts. Avascular surfaces, such as bone without periosteum or cartilage without perichondrium, cannot support an overlying full-thickness graft, which will lead to graft failure. A delayed closure is sometimes preferred to immediate reconstruction, as it allows for improved vascularity of the bed.[22] Additionally, subcutaneous adipose tissue is poorly vascularized, so skin grafts need to be defatted after harvesting.

In addition to epidermal sutures, full-thickness skin grafts are usually immobilized and secured in place using a basting suture or a tie-over bolster dressing. This technique improves adhesion of the graft to its recipient bed, reduces potential dead space, and helps prevent hematoma or seroma formation.[23]

For young or active patients with defects on the trunk or extremities, heterografts, such as porcine xenografts or artificial skin equivalents, allow for more rapid return to activity than surgical repair does. The xenograft acts as a biological dressing and allows for increased comfort during healing by second intent.[24] It dissolves over the course of 1–2 weeks. The drawback is that healing takes longer than with surgical closure, but the end result is often a smaller, less noticeable scar. Xenografts can even be used with success on large defects of the genitalia that do not penetrate the fascia when surgical repair would otherwise distort the anatomy and compromise function (Figure 2.12).

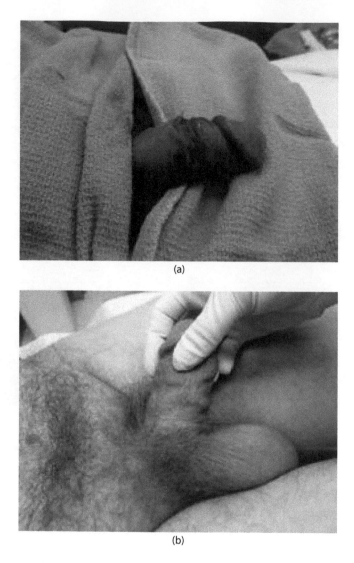

(a)

(b)

FIGURE 2.12   Porcine xenografts can be used for large defects on the genitalia with preservation of function and cosmesis. (a) Xenograft sutured in place following removal of a large squamous cell carcinoma in situ on the penis. (b) Appearance at 2-month follow-up, with acceptable cosmesis and preservation of function, considering the size of the original surgical defect.

Postoperative Management

Postoperative management is just as critical in optimizing outcome as intraoperative techniques. Caring for a postoperative wound can seem daunting to patients and caregivers. Patients who are unsure of appropriate wound care are more vulnerable to infection and desiccation. In turn, healing time may be prolonged and aesthetic appearance may be compromised. Thus, thorough wound care instructions given in both oral and written form, preferably in the presence of family members, are essential.

In addition to wound care, the instructions should discuss likely or anticipated sequelae, as well as how to recognize the most common complications and how the patient should initially manage them. Contact information for the person on call should also be provided.

Though a variety of topical agents and dressing materials with different characteristics have been used by dermatological surgeons, in our practice, a petrolatum-based ointment and a nonadhesive dressing are applied to the wound immediately after surgery, followed by a pressure dressing to reduce the risk for bleeding. This dressing can be changed by the patient to a lighter dressing, as appropriate, within 24–48 hours. Though topical antibacterial agents have traditionally been used for fresh cutaneous wounds, recent studies suggest they have no advantage over plain petrolatum-based ointments. In addition, topical antibacterial agents may cause allergic contact dermatitis.[25,26]

Traditionally, sutures are removed 5–7 days after placement on the face, 7–10 days on the neck, and 10–14 days on the scalp, trunk, and extremities. However, sutures can be left in place longer in elderly patients, given their increased epidermal regeneration time. For example, sutures may remain for up to 10 days on the face to allow for adequate healing in this population.

CONCLUSIONS

Proper planning and surgical technique are critical to the success of cutaneous reconstruction. When feasible, a simpler approach can result in significantly fewer postoperative complications, faster healing, and greater satisfaction for both the surgeon and the patient. Often less is more. Refinement of repairs in the postoperative period can further optimize long-term appearance. Techniques such as surgical scar revision, dermabrasion, laser surgery, and intralesional injections can be utilized to improve scar cosmesis and will be addressed in Part II of this book.

REFERENCES

1. Walker J. What is the effect of preoperative information on patient satisfaction? *Br J Nurs* 2007;16(1):27–32.
2. Vachiramon V, Sobanko J, Rattanaumpawan P, Miller C. Music reduces patient anxiety during Mohs surgery: An open-label randomized controlled trial. *Dermatol Surg* 2013;39(2):298–305.
3. Rudin D, Kiss A, Wetz R, Sottile V. Music in the endoscopy suite: A meta-analysis of randomized controlled studies. *Endosc* 2007;39(6):507–10.
4. Fosko SW, Gibney MD, Harrison B. Repetitive pinching of the skin during lidocaine infiltration reduces patient discomfort. *J Am Acad Dermatol* 1998;39(1):74–8.
5. Marcus BC. Wound closure techniques. In: Baker S (ed). *Local Flaps in Facial Reconstruction,* 2nd ed. Philadelphia: Mosby; 2007, pp. 41–7.
6. Fincher EF, Gladstone HB, Moy RL. Complex layered facial closures. In: Robinson JK, Hanke CW, Siegel DM, Fratila A (eds). *Surgery of the Skin*, 2nd ed. Philadelphia: Mosby; 2010, pp. 212–3.
7. Weitzul S, Taylor RS. Suturing materials and epidermal closure techniques. In: Robinson JK, Hanke CW, Siegel DM, Fratila A (eds). *Surgery of the Skin*. 2nd ed. Philadelphia: Mosby; 2010, pp. 190.
8. Tierney E, Kouba D. A subcutaneous corset plication rapidly and effectively relieves tension on large linear closures. *Dermatol Surg* 2009;35(11):1806–8.
9. Sebben JE. Electrosurgery principles: Cutting current and cutaneous surgery—Part I. *J Dermatol Surg Oncol* 1988;14(1):29-31.
10. Hainer B. Electrosurgery for the skin. *Am Fam Physician* 2002;66(7):1259–66.

11. Soon SL, Washington CV, Jr. Electrosurgery, electrocoagulation, electrofulguration, electrodesiccation, electrosection, electrocautery. In: Robinson JK, Hanke CW, Siegel DM, Fratila A (eds). *Surgery of the Skin*. 2nd ed. Philadelphia: Mosby; 2010, pp. 143–4.
12. Lenzy Y, Cummins D, Finn D. Bipolar forceps: A hemostatic tool for patients with electrocoagulation-induced dental pain. *J Am Acad Dermatol* 2011;65(2):441–2.
13. Rohrer T. Planning the closure. *Semin Cutan Med Surg* 2003;22(4):244–54.
14. Donaldson M, Coldiron B. Scars after second intention healing. *Facial Plast Surg* 2012;28(5): 497–503.
15. Zitelli J. Secondary intention healing: An alternative to surgical repair. *Clin Dermatol* 1984;2(3):92-105.
16. Mott K, Clark D, Stelljes L. Regional variation in wound contraction of Mohs surgery defects allowed to heal by second intention. *Dermatol Surg* 2003;29(7):712–22.
17. Zitelli J. Wound healing by secondary intention: A cosmetic appraisal. *J Am Acad Dermatol* 1983;9(3):407-15.
18. Campbell R, Perlis C, Malik M, Dufresne R. Characteristics of Mohs practices in the United States: A recall survey of ACMS surgeons. *Dermatol Surg* 2007;33(12):1413–8.
19. Soliman S, Hatef D, Hollier L, Thornton J. The rationale for direct linear closure of facial Mohs' defects. *Plastic Reconstr Surg* 2011;127(1):142–9.
20. Moody B, McCarthy J, Linder J, Hruza G. Enhanced cosmetic outcome with running horizontal mattress sutures. *Dermatol Surg* 2005;31(10):1313–6.
21. Rapstine E, Knaus W, Thornton J. Simplifying cheek reconstruction: A review of over 400 cases. *Plastic Reconstr Surg* 2012;129(6):1291–9.
22. Thibault MJ, Bennett RG. Success of delayed full-thickness skin grafts after Mohs micrographic surgery. *J Am Acad Dermatol* 1995;32(6):1004–9.
23. Hill TG. Enhancing the survival of full-thickness grafts. *J Dermatol Surg Oncol* 1984;10(8):639–42.
24. Prystowsky J, Siegel D, Ascherman J. Artificial skin for closure of wounds created by skin cancer excisions. *Dermatol Surg* 2001;27(7):648–54.
25. Campbell RM, Perlis CS, Fisher E, Gloster HM, Jr. Gentamicin ointment versus petrolatum for management of auricular wounds. *Dermatol Surg* 2005;31(6):664–9.
26. Draelos ZD, Rizer RL, Trookman NS. A comparison of postprocedural wound care treatments: Do antibiotic-based ointments improve outcomes? *J Am Acad Dermatol* 2011;64 Suppl 3:S23–S29.

Chapter 3

Intraoperative Surgical Techniques and Pearls—Special Considerations

Matteo C. LoPiccolo and Thomas E. Rohrer

INTRODUCTION

This chapter is intended to provide the reconstructive surgeon with a set of surgical pearls and techniques that are applicable to closing defects in unique areas of skin. A comprehensive discussion of defect types and repair options for these sites is beyond the scope of this chapter. Instead, the fundamental principles that are applicable to a variety of reconstructive strategies are presented, with the aim of maximizing aesthetic and functional outcomes.

EYELIDS

The primary purpose of the eyelid is to protect the globe and to maintain a moist environment for the cornea. The principal goal in repairing defects of the lid and periorbital tissue is to fully restore these functions as well as to achieve a pleasing aesthetic outcome. Knowledge of lid anatomy is paramount to successfully accomplish these goals. It is useful for the surgeon to consider the eyelid as composed of posterior, middle, and anterior lamellae (Figure 3.1). The posterior lamella is the portion of the eyelid closest to the globe. It is composed of the conjunctiva that covers the inner surface of the lid and is continuous with that of the globe. The middle lamella consists of the firm connective tissue of the tarsal plate, as well as lid retractors and the orbital septum. The tarsus is important for providing structure and form to the lids. The anterior lamella comprises the pretarsal portion of the palpebral orbicularis oculi muscle and a thin layer of skin covering the anterior surface of the lid. The division between the anterior and posterior lamellae is demarcated along the lid margin by the gray line. This structure lies posterior to the lash line and anterior to the orifices of the Meibomian glands. It is important for the surgeon to visualize the gray line to ensure proper alignment during lid reconstruction (Figure 3.2).

The lacrimal gland resides in the postseptal space lateral to the supraorbital fat pads. Tears originate from this gland to lubricate the conjunctiva and ultimately collect into the upper and lower lacrimal punctae at the medial eyelid margins. The lacrimal punctae continue medially to form the superior and inferior canaliculi, which lead to the lacrimal sac, located posterior to the medial canthal tendon. The lacrimal sac drains into the nasolacrimal duct and ultimately into the inferior nasal turbinate (Figure 3.3).[1]

When approaching a defect of the eyelid, its depth, width, and the extent to which it involves critical lid structures must be assessed. Defects involving only the anterior lamella may be closed in a linear fashion, with a cutaneous or myocutaneous flap, or using a partial- or full-thickness skin graft. Regardless of the strategy, care must be taken to ensure that the

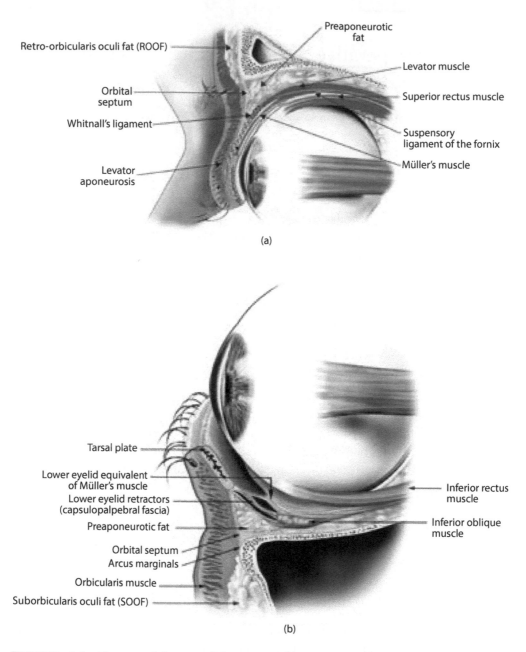

FIGURE 3.1 Upper and lower eyelid anatomy. (a) Upper eyelid. (b) Lower eyelid. (From Leatherbarrow, B., *Oculoplastic Surgery,* 2nd ed., London, Informa Healthcare, 2011.)

tension vector is oriented perpendicular to the lid margin. The lid should be undermined in the pretarsal plane; the undermining may be extended onto the cheek in the subcutaneous layer.[2] This is often useful during the planning phase to more accurately assess tissue laxity. Undermining should be performed until little to no tension remains at the wound edges. When sufficient tissue has been freed, anchoring sutures are placed from the underside of the flap to the periosteum of the orbital rim to support flap position and to reduce tension.

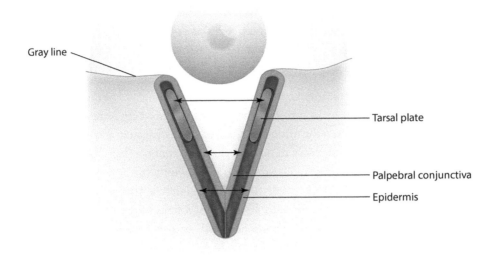

FIGURE 3.2   Aligning of gray line during eyelid reconstruction.

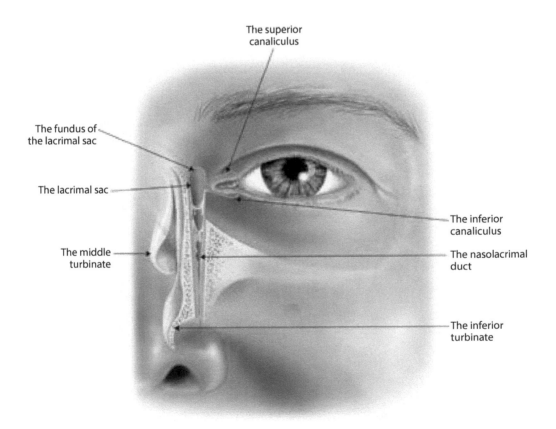

FIGURE 3.3   The lacrimal drainage system. (From Leatherbarrow, B., *Oculoplastic Surgery,* 2nd ed., London, Informa Healthcare, 2011.)

This strategy may also be employed when executing a linear repair in a patient with a high risk for ectropion, to guard against lid contraction.[2] This is often useful during the planning phase option, the upper lid is an excellent source of donor skin. When upper lid laxity is not sufficient to support a graft harvest, pre- or postauricular skin may also be used.

The approach to the repair of full-thickness lid defects is often thought to be dictated by the percentage of the lid skin involved in the defect. Lid behavior varies, however, from patient to patient, and selecting the proper strategy for reconstruction rests on adequately assessing lid tension.[2] A small defect that is closed primarily in one patient may require a flap repair in another. A stepwise approach should be taken to relieve wound tension until the lid margin may be easily approximated. A simple layered side-to-side closure should first be attempted. If sufficient tension exists to prevent closure, a lateral cantholysis or canthotomy may be performed. The conjunctiva just inferior to the lateral canthus may be bluntly dissected along the periosteum until the lateral canthal tendon is identified (Figure 3.4). Release of this tendon alone may provide sufficient movement to perform lid closure. If needed, a canthotomy incision placed through the lateral canthus and angled superiorly at roughly 30 degrees will further decrease tension.

In cases where additional release is needed, the canthotomy incision may be extended in a semicircle superiorly and laterally to develop a Tenzel flap.[3] This myocutaneous flap should be undermined just under the orbicularis oculi until sufficient mobility has been achieved to allow apposition of the lid margin. Anchoring sutures should then be placed from the undersurface of the flap to the lateral orbital rim. Repair of large defects of the lid margin may be accomplished with this procedure.

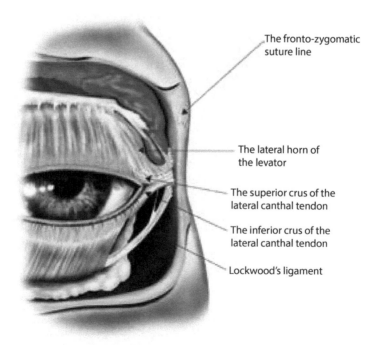

The fronto-zygomatic suture line

The lateral horn of the levator

The superior crus of the lateral canthal tendon

The inferior crus of the lateral canthal tendon

Lockwood's ligament

FIGURE 3.4   The lateral canthal tendon. (From Leatherbarrow, B., *Oculoplastic Surgery*, 2nd ed., London, Informa Healthcare, 2011.)

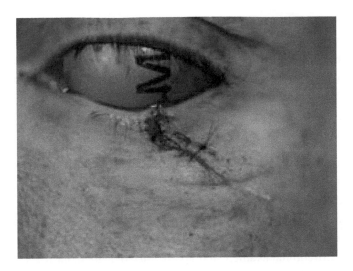

FIGURE 3.5 Eyelid wound closed with Vicryl suture. Care is taken to align the lid margin. The suture is left long and then tucked under subsequent sutures to keep it from abrading the cornea.

Once tension has been alleviated, the lid may be repaired. The posterior lamella is approximated first, by placing a vertical mattress suture through the lid margin and the tarsal plate. The gray line should be used as a guide to ensure proper alignment of the wound edges, and careful attention should be paid to eversion of the margin to avoid notching.

A soft, braided suture material such as 6-0 polyglactin 910 (Vicryl, Ethicon Endosurgery, Inc., Somerville, NJ) should be used in the posterior lamella to minimize corneal irritation and to maximize patient comfort. Upon tying the knot for this stitch, the authors prefer to cut the suture long and keep it draped away from the cornea. The superficial layer of sutures is later run over the top of the excess Vicryl, holding it in place against the epidermis and away from the lid margin (Figure 3.5). This greatly reduces the risk of corneal injury in the postoperative period. Following repair of the posterior lamella, buried sutures are then placed to close the dermis and muscular layer of the anterior lamella. One must be aware of the orientation of the eyelashes during this step, making sure they are angled away from the globe equally on both sides of the lid. Finally, superficial sutures are used to align the epidermis.

LIPS

The lip is a complex anatomic structure important for word formation, eating, kissing, and facial expression. Analogous to the case of the eyelid, restoration of these functions is the primary goal of lip reconstruction. The perioral skin is also a center of aesthetic attraction, and achieving a pleasing cosmetic result is of near equally importance. A variety of reconstructive options may be employed in this region, depending on the location and extent of the defect. A general set of pearls and concepts are presented here to aid the surgeon in achieving optimal results in a variety of reconstructive designs.

When planning repairs in this area, careful attention should be paid to the unique surface anatomy of the region. The upper cutaneous lip is demarcated superiorly by the nasal sill, laterally by the melolabial folds, and inferiorly by the vermilion border and is divided into three separate subunits by the philtral columns. The lower cutaneous lip is a single subunit demarcated by the labiomental crease, the melolabial folds, and the lower vermilion border. The vermilion comprises the fifth perioral subunit (Figure 3.6). These individual units should be considered when designing repairs, and each unit should be reconstructed separately, if possible.[4] It is also beneficial to place incisions along the anatomical features demarcating these units, which provide excellent camouflage for scar lines.

The perioral tissue swells significantly with manipulation and infiltration of local anesthetic, so the subunits should be outlined with a surgical marking pen prior to the first injection. Regional nerve blocks will also help to minimize the distortion of these landmarks. For the upper lip, an infraorbital nerve block may be attained through an intraoral approach by inserting a needle though the superior labial sulcus just above the canine (Figure 3.7). The needle is then advanced 1 cm toward the infraorbital foramen, and approximately 1 mL of local anesthetic is injected. Similarly, for the lower lip, a mental nerve block is performed by advancing a needle several millimeters through the inferior labial sulcus between the first and second premolars, angled toward the mental foramen.[5] Again, approximately 1 mL of local anesthetic is injected at this location.

When evaluating a lip defect, an attempt to re-approximate the wound edges with skin hooks should first be made to assess the degree of tension. Vertical incision lines blend well in the perioral region, even when crossing the vermilion, and primary closure is often an excellent option. In fact, a linear closure is often possible for defects involving nearly 50% of the surface area of the lip and a wedge excision can typically yield excellent aesthetic and functional results in such cases. Undermining just above the orbicularis oris muscle may facilitate a great deal of tissue movement. In addition, in the event a mucosal advancement is needed, one should dissect below the level of the minor salivary glands.

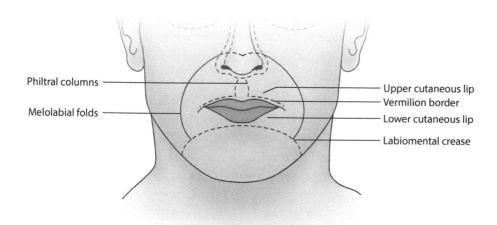

FIGURE 3.6   Cosmetic subunits of the perioral area.

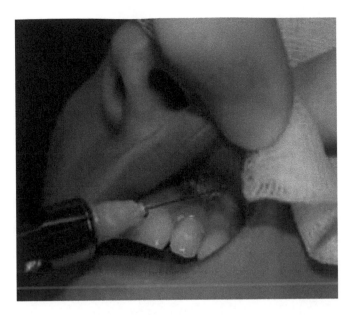

FIGURE 3.7   Infraorbital nerve block to anesthetize the upper lip.

A variety of laterally based advancement flaps may be elevated along the upper or lower lip to facilitate closure of large defects not amenable to side-to-side closure. Though a variety of complex flaps have been described in literature,[6] often smaller rotation or advancement flaps offer excellent aesthetic results and are more tolerable for the patient (Figure 3.8). If necessary, wide undermining of the cheek may be performed to increase tissue movement, and periosteal tacking sutures may then be placed to recreate the melolabial fold.[5]

For a full-thickness defect of the lip, the mucosal, muscular, dermal, and epidermal layers should be repaired individually for optimal results (Figure 3.9). A soft, braided, absorbable suture, such as Vicryl, should be used to close the intraoral mucosa, and the knot should be tied internally just beneath the muscular layer. The orbicularis oris is repaired next; it must be fully approximated to restore function to the oral aperture. When closing the cutaneous layer, care must be taken to accurately align the vermilion border to avoid mismatch or notching. This is of the utmost importance. In instances where ink lines become smudged and a scalpel mark has not been placed, the white roll of the lip can guide alignment.[7] The dermis and epidermis of the vermilion may be closed with a single layer of suture, and the vertical mattress technique may be used to encourage wound eversion.

As the lip experiences repetitive stress in the postoperative period, the delicate mucosa has a tendency to tear around superficial sutures. As opposed to finer monofilaments, braided sutures tend to be softer and less traumatic, with silk being the traditional choice of many surgeons for mucosal closures.[8] While an excellent option for the mucosa, silk is not commonly used for deep or superficial repair of the cutaneous lip; this necessitates a third suture type for a single closure. Vicryl is commonly utilized to approximate the deeper layers in lip reconstruction, and the authors find that it provides comfort, function, and cosmetic results equivalent to those of silk in the repair of the superficial mucosa. Using this alternative can help minimize the use of resources when repairing defects of the mucosal lip.

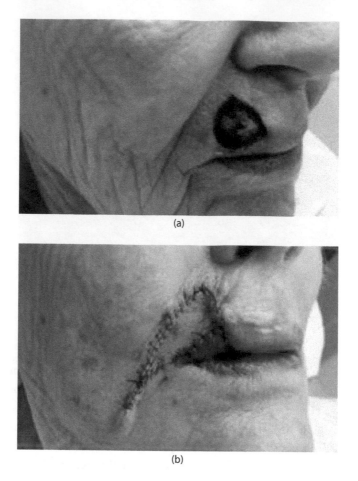

(a)

(b)

FIGURE 3.8   A V-Y advancement flap and mucosal advancement to repair a large defect involving both the cutaneous and the vermilion upper lip. (a) Before the repair. (b) Immediately after the repair. (Courtesy of Alexander L. Berlin, MD.)

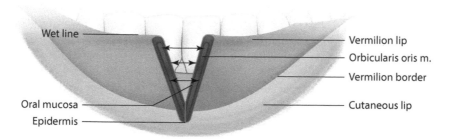

FIGURE 3.9   Full-thickness repair of the lip involves separate repair of the individual layers that compose the lip.

SCALP AND EXTREMITIES

Scalp and extremity wounds may present a unique set of reconstructive challenges, such as relatively low tissue laxity, high skin tension, and reduced circulation, especially in the lower extremities of older patients. Prior to designing any closure at these locations, the degree of tissue laxity surrounding the defect should be assessed by simply squeezing the sides of the wound together.

In cases where the tissue affords no laxity, one may allow defects to granulate with reasonably good results. Scalp defects involving the deep dermis that are surrounded by terminal hair growth will likely benefit from a flap repair to eliminate focal alopecia. A rotation flap is commonly employed and helps to offset the relative inelasticity of skin at this location. In contrast, defects that do not extend below the level of the hair bulb often regrow hair when allowed to granulate. In these instances, large flap or graft repairs for scalp or extremity defects may not be necessary, as second intent healing often affords equivalent or superior results with less morbidity.

When some degree of tissue laxity exists but complete closure is not possible, the authors commonly employ a purse string closure to decrease wound surface area and, consequently, healing time.[9] The surface area of most wounds of the scalp and extremities can be reduced to some degree by using a purse string closure. An absorbable suture, such as Vicryl or poligle-caprone 25 (Monocryl, Ethicon Endosurgery, Inc., Somerville, NJ), is ideal. Additional deep sutures may be placed to align the wound in the optimal direction of closure or to partially close the lateral portions of the defect. Undermining generally is of little help in reducing wound diameter with a partial purse string closure. Moreover, it may increase the risk of bleeding in a patient with a partially open defect and is therefore avoided by the authors.

In cases where sufficient laxity exists, complete closure of the defect should be performed. Though many extremity defects can be closed linearly, the surgeon should carefully assess the patient before excising an ellipse. In areas of repetitive motion, such as the shoulder, especially in young or muscular patients with high skin tension, even the most carefully performed elliptical closure may result in a widened, "fish-mouth" scar with time. These patients may be best served by using a purse string suture for a complete closure. This option produces many small standing tissue cones at the periphery of the defect and may appear less elegant at the time of repair. Tension and repetitive motion reliably reduce these cones, however, and the long-term result is a shorter and often thinner scar than that which would result from a traditional linear ellipse.[9] In the instance where a purse string alone is not sufficient for achieving complete closure, additional deep sutures may be used to fully approximate the wound edges in a modified purse string repair[10] (Figure 3.10).

When properly selected, a traditional linear closure may be used for many extremity and scalp defects. For extremity defects, the authors recommend wide undermining in the layer of the superficial fat to decrease tension and minimize scar width. Extremity defects extending to the fascia, such as those following melanoma extirpations, are afforded ample movement along the fascial plane without the need for further undermining. As described in Chapter 2, fascial plication sutures are of benefit in reducing wound tension in these

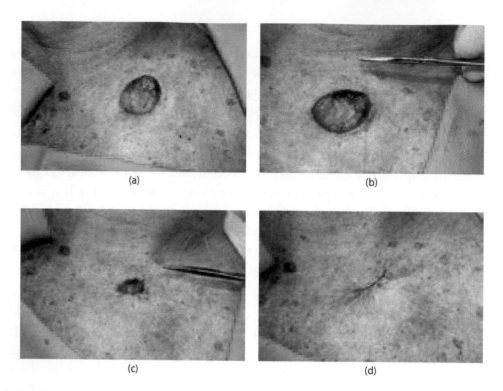

(a)   (b)

(c)   (d)

FIGURE 3.10   Modified purse string closure. In the instance where a purse string alone is not sufficient at achieving complete closure, additional deep sutures may be used to accomplish full approximation of the wound edges in a modified purse string repair. (a) Wound following Mohs surgery. (b) A purse string suture is placed around the wound. (c) The suture is drawn tight to reduce the diameter of the wound. (d) Additional sutures are placed across the wound to close it down further.

instances and should be placed prior to approximation of the dermis. Extremity skin is subject to increased tension and motion, as well as a less robust blood supply than the face. The time needed for healing is thus often increased, as is the risk of track mark scarring from superficial sutures. To avoid this, a running subcuticular stitch may be used for epidermal approximation (Figure 3.11). These sutures can remain in place for 2 to 3 weeks, if necessary, without leaving significant track marks.

Extremity wounds near joints require additional considerations due to the risk of joint contracture and the consequent reduced range of motion. Whenever possible, linear closures should be oriented in such a way as not to cross joint lines. S-plasty and Z-plasty can be used to lengthen and reorient the final scar and to minimize the risk of contracture.

When excising an ellipse on hair-bearing scalp, the scalpel blade should be directed at an angle parallel to the direction of the follicles. This helps to minimize trauma to the hair bulbs, thus limiting postoperative alopecia. For the same reason, the use of electrocautery should be limited. Scalp defects should be extended to the depth of the subgalea, as the loose areolar tissue of this layer is relatively avascular and provides an ideal plane in which to undermine (Figure 3.12). Extensive undermining, however, often yields only a small gain in tissue movement on the scalp. Care should be taken to re-approximate the galea in order to prevent inversion and spread of the final scar line. In addition, the galea is best sutured separately from the dermis.[11]

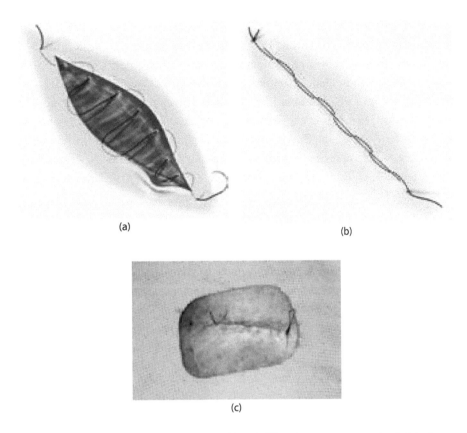

(a)

(b)

(c)

FIGURE 3.11   Running subcuticular suture. (a) and (b) When sutures must be left in longer than a week, a running subcuticular stitch may be utilized to prevent suture marks. (c) Completed suture. (From Leatherbarrow, B., *Oculoplastic Surgery,* 2nd ed., London, Informa Healthcare, 2011.)

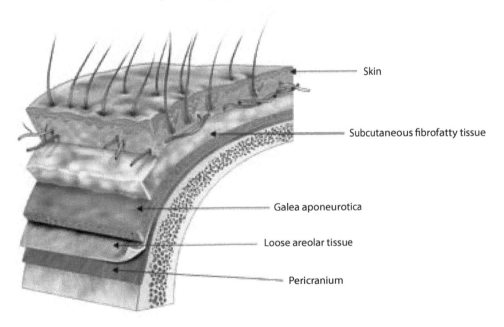

Skin

Subcutaneous fibrofatty tissue

Galea aponeurotica

Loose areolar tissue

Pericranium

FIGURE 3.12   Tissue layers in central scalp (From Leatherbarrow, B., *Oculoplastic Surgery,* 2nd ed., London, Informa Healthcare, 2011.)

Wound care in scalp and extremity repairs is of the utmost importance, especially in wounds allowed to heal by secondary intention. Educating the patient or caregiver is critical, as several weeks to months may be necessary for complete healing of larger surgical defects. Frequent follow-up visits may be needed for patient reassurance, and home nursing care should be considered for patients who are unable to perform dressing changes. In addition, patients with lower extremity wounds in the setting of poor circulation or edema may benefit from the placement of an Unna boot. This compression dressing consists of a two-layered circumferential wrap: a gauze impregnated with zinc oxide, followed by an elastic wrap, such as ACE elastic bandage (3M, St. Paul, MN) or Coban (3M, St. Paul, MN). The Unna boot can be left in place for up to 1 week at a time.

CONCLUSIONS

Although the general surgical techniques described in Chapter 2 also apply to repairs at the locations discussed in this chapter, knowledge of the local anatomy and specific characteristics of the eyelids, lips, scalp, and extremities is critical to proper repair. These specific techniques should help the surgeon to achieve the most functional and most cosmetically pleasing final result.

REFERENCES

1. Salasche S. Anatomy. In: Rohrer T, Cook JL, Nguyen T, Mellette JR (eds). *Flaps and Grafts in Dermatologic Surgery*. Philadelphia: Elsevier; 2007.
2. Nerad J. Eyelid reconstruction. In: *Techniques in Ophthalmic Plastic Surgery: A Personal Tutorial*. Philadelphia: Elsevier; 2012.
3. Tenzel RR, Stewart WB. Eyelid reconstruction by the semicircle flap technique. *Ophthalmology* 1978;85(11):1164–9.
4. Zitelli JA, Brodland DG. A regional approach to reconstruction of the upper lip. *J Dermatol Surg Oncol* 1991;17(2):143–8.
5. Chapman JT, Mellette JR. Perioral reconstruction. In: Rohrer T, Cook JL, Nguyen T, Mellette JR (eds). *Flaps and Grafts in Dermatologic Surgery*. Philadelphia: Elsevier; 2007.
6. Ebrahimi A, Maghsoudnia GR, Arshadi AA. Prospective comparative study of lower lip defects reconstruction with different local flaps. *J Craniofac Surg* 2011;22(6):2255–9.
7. LoPiccolo MC, Kouba DJ. Bilateral eri-alar advancement flap to close a midline upper lip defect. *Dermatol Surg* 2011;37(8):1159–62.
8. Huang CC, Arpey CJ. The lips: Excision and repair. *Dermatol Clin* 1998;16:127–43.
9. Tremolada C, Blandini D, Beretta M, Mascetti M. The "round block" purse-string suture: A simple method to close skin defects with minimal scarring. *Plastic Reconstr Surg* 1997;100(1):126–31.
10. Hoffman A, Lander J, Lee PK. Modification of the purse-string closure for large defects of the extremities. *Dermatol Surg* 2008;34(2):243–5.
11. Lee KK, Mehrany K, Swanson NA. Scalp reconstruction. In: Rohrer T, Cook JL, Nguyen T, Mellette JR (eds). *Flaps and Grafts in Dermatologic Surgery*. Philadelphia: Elsevier; 2007.

Chapter 4

Complications in Mohs Surgery

Jordan B. Slutsky and Scott W. Fosko

INTRODUCTION

Even with appropriate patient selection, careful surgical planning, and meticulous surgical technique, complications can occur during and after Mohs micrographic surgery and wound reconstruction. Thankfully, the complication rates for Mohs surgery are low and studies have consistently demonstrated the safety of Mohs in the outpatient setting, even in the nonagenarian population.[1,2,3] Knowledge of potential complications, a focus on prevention and early detection, and appropriate management are paramount. This chapter reviews complications as they may occur during and after Mohs surgery in chronological order. The focus is on surgery of the head and neck, given the highest rates of Mohs at these sites.

PREOPERATIVE PERIOD
Time-Outs and Checklists

Time-outs are standard practice in operating rooms and are used to confirm patient, surgical site, and allergies prior to incision. In the Mohs setting, time-outs can be used in conjunction with surgical checklists to ensure accurate and safe surgery.

Numerous studies have demonstrated that checklists are an economical and effective method of enhancing patient safety in the surgical setting by decreasing morbidity and mortality.[4,5,6] Surgical checklists are so important that they are the focus of the World Health Organization (WHO)'s second Global Patient Safety Challenge and its publication *WHO Guidelines for Safe Surgery: Safe Surgery Saves Lives*.[7,8] The WHO checklist is intended for use in the operating room, which is very similar to the Mohs surgery environment, and is modeled on the checklists used for over 70 years in the aviation industry, which has an excellent track record of safety.

Although we are not aware of any studies specifically examining their use in Mohs surgery, checklists can be tailored to one's own workflow and processes to enhance patient safety and to ensure accurate surgical documentation. Mohs checklists may include patient identifiers, such as name, date of birth, and address; tumor-specific information, such as site and tumor type; and patient information, such as allergies, anticoagulant medications and supplements, need for antibiotics, antivirals, or sterile trays, known communicable disease, implanted electronic devices, and tobacco or alcohol use. Important components of a Mohs checklist are areas to indicate that consent has been signed, that the site has been confirmed by the patient, and that a preoperative photograph (as well as subsequent photographs documenting defect and repair) has been taken. Perhaps the most important part of an effective Mohs checklist is an area for the Mohs surgeon and staff to initial prior to commencing each stage or repair to ensure that the correct patient is in the surgical chair. The authors have found it important to have at least two members of the Mohs team double-check the checklist to ensure accuracy and patient safety.

An important consideration with checklists is that they are effective only when used correctly. One study found 100% association of preincision utilization with subsequent decreased use of individual checkpoints;[9] in other words, checklists are helpful only when Mohs surgeons and their staff use them diligently, consistently, and accurately. This is consistent with the authors' experience that staff focus is often sharpest at the start of a Mohs day and there can be staff drift as the day proceeds and variables are introduced. Occasionally auditing the checklists to make sure they are being utilized correctly is important.

An emerging challenge in health care is the migration away from paper charting to electronic documentation. In the senior author's opinion, this change is "transformational" in many ways and its impact on documentation, accuracy, and ultimately patient safety remains to be fully understood.

Wrong-Site Surgery

The first potential complication to be avoided is operating on the wrong surgical site, the most common sentinel event in all of medicine reported to the Joint Commission in the United States. Data on wrong-site surgery in Mohs is limited, but a study found 14% of malpractice cases involving Mohs surgeons were the result of wrong-site surgery.[10] Many Mohs patients are referred after a biopsy by a general dermatologist or primary care physician; in such cases, the Mohs surgeon is not familiar with the biopsy site. Factors that can make site identification difficult include healing of the biopsy site; other scars from prior biopsies, surgeries, or cryotherapy; and actinic damage (Figure 4.1).

Studies have found that between 9% and 16.6% of patients are unable to correctly identify the biopsy site.[11,12] One study, which found that patients incorrectly identified the biopsy site in 16.6% of cases, also found that the physician incorrectly identified the biopsy site in 5.9% of cases and that the physician and the patient both incorrectly identified the site in 4.4% of cases. Interestingly, one patient in this study disagreed on the biopsy site, despite being shown

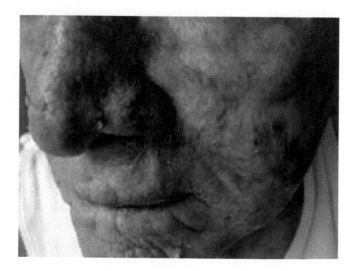

FIGURE 4.1   Elderly patient with numerous scars, actinic damage, and multiple suspicious lesions, making identification of healed biopsy site difficult.

a photograph from the day of the biopsy with the needle injecting the site.[12] This highlights the fact that while patient confirmation is an important step in proper site identification, even the most confident patients can provide incorrect information. Our aging population and the possible associated decline in cognitive skills will only add to this challenge.

Photographs are the most useful documentation to decrease the risk for wrong-site surgery; ideally, they should have the lesion circled, be in focus, and include nearby anatomic reference points.[10] Two photographs are helpful: one "pulled back" to include nearby landmarks and another close up, showing local lesions and surface changes.[12] When there is uncertainty about site identification and no photos are available, the authors circle and photograph the suspected biopsy site during their consultation and send the picture to the referring physician for confirmation. Patients may also take photos of lesions of concern before or after a biopsy; this may be an additional safeguard in regard to site identification that our patients can actively contribute to. The authors also find it helpful to have family members who may be familiar with the biopsy site confirm its location.

Diagrams of the biopsy site with distance measurements from nearby fixed anatomic landmarks (i.e., triangulation) can also be used in addition to or in lieu of photographs.[13] The authors have found dermoscopy a useful tool to identify subtle signs of residual tumor or biopsy scars. Gauze dermabrasion may reveal recent biopsy sites to be more friable than surrounding skin.[12] Wood's light examination may reveal dyspigmentation of a recent biopsy site, and one study demonstrated that an ultraviolet-fluorescent tattoo at the time of biopsy can help surgeons identify the site with Wood's light at a later time.[14]

Patient Anxiety and Movement

A unique aspect of Mohs surgery is the ability to treat cutaneous malignancies in the office with the use of local anesthetics. The vast majority of Mohs patients are awake during surgery, and many of them are anxious. Several techniques, including proper positioning and lighting, administration of anxiolytics, and use of distractions during surgery, have been found to be very effective in alleviating anxiety, as described in Chapter 2. In addition, many Mohs surgeons, including the authors, use surgical towels or drapes to isolate the surgical field and block the bright glare of surgical lights. Most patients are fine with being draped intraoperatively, but some may complain of claustrophobia. Whenever possible, care should be taken to leave the nostrils and mouth uncovered for ease of breathing.

Mohs patients must be made aware that movement may compromise their safety as well as the safety of the Mohs team. The authors ask their patients to keep their hands out of the surgical field and to let the Mohs team know if they need to move, cough, or sneeze intraoperatively. Additional causes of patient movement include shivering, if the surgical suite is cold, and intrinsic trembling, such as essential tremor or Parkinson's disease.

Reactions to Antiseptics and Anesthetics

Commonly used antiseptics in Mohs surgery include betadine and chlorhexidine. Though generally safe in cutaneous surgery, betadine can cause either irritant or allergic contact dermatitis, while chlorhexidine can cause corneal toxicity on contact with the eye or ototox-icity on contact with the inner ear (in patients with a perforated tympanic membrane).[15,16]

Local anesthetics are divided into two classes: amides, such as lidocaine, bupivacaine, and prilocaine, and esters, such as benzocaine, procaine, and tetracaine. The amide lidocaine is the most commonly used local anesthetic in Mohs surgery, usually at the dose of 1% with 1:100,000 epinephrine. Lidocaine dosing is weight based (maximum 7mg/kg when mixed with epineph-rine, 4.5mg/kg without epinephrine), and toxicity is rare with Mohs surgery. Early signs of lidocaine toxicity correspond to blood levels of 1–5 µg/mL and include increased anxiety, talk-ativeness, tinnitus, perioral or tongue tingling and numbness, nausea and vomiting, metallic taste, and double vision. Early toxicity is best managed with recognition of toxicity, discontinua-tion of further anesthetic use, and observation. Nystagmus, muscle twitching, and tremors indi-cate midrange toxicity (5–8 µg/mL), and the need to admit the patient for hospital observation. Blood levels of 8–12 µg/mL can result in seizures and respiratory arrest, for which emergency medical services (EMS) should be contacted while establishing an airway and administering oxygen. Benzodiazepines, such as lorazepam or diazepam, may be given for seizures.[17]

Amides are metabolized by the liver and should be used with caution in patients with liver disease. Allergy to lidocaine is rare and can be due to hypersensitivity to either lidocaine or its preservatives (parabens or sulfites).[17]

Epinephrine added to lidocaine prolongs the duration of anesthesia and helps with hemo-stasis via vasoconstriction. A recent study found 25 minutes to be the optimal time delay between injection of epinephrine and incision to minimize bleeding, based on spectroscopic measurements of soft tissue hemoglobin concentration.[18] The authors often have a patient wait after administration of anesthesia with lidocaine/epinephrine for maximum hemostasis while attending to other patients.

Epinephrine can cause tachycardia and uneasiness in some patients. The senior author has observed that patients may experience the sensation of a rapid heartbeat but without objective tachycardia on pulse monitoring. Diluting lidocaine/epinephrine anesthetic to half strength with sterile saline can minimize side effects without affecting efficacy, and the authors often use this technique for large tumors requiring high volumes of anesthetic, similar to tumescent anesthesia.

Other local anesthetics used in Mohs include bupivacaine, which has a longer duration of action but also a longer onset of action than lidocaine; side effects include cardiotoxicity at high doses. Some surgeons add bupivacaine to their lidocaine solution to extend the duration of anesthesia.

Care should be taken to avoid injecting anesthetic directly into a vessel or a crucial structure such as the globe. In addition, local anesthetics can cause temporary paralysis and paresis when infiltrated adjacent to motor nerves. Local tissue edema can also result from the injec-tion of local anesthesia. These complications will be discussed in the section "Nerve Trauma."

It is prudent to review the recommended dosages and potential side effects of local anesthetics prior to their use and to have oxygen and benzodiazepines available in case of emergencies. Lidocaine is pregnancy category B, whereas epinephrine and bupivacaine are category C.

Vasovagal Syncope

Vasovagal reactions can occur at any point during Mohs surgery but can happen as early as site confirmation or local anesthesia. Predisposed patients will often have a history of fainting; such responses may be triggered by stress or the sight of blood. Vasovagal syncope is characterized by hypotension, bradycardia, and sometimes brief loss of consciousness. Patients may exhibit pallor and diaphoresis, in which case they should be immediately reclined in the supine or Trendelenburg position to maximize blood flow to the brain. Cool compresses, drinks, and snacks can be given while vitals are monitored and patients recuperate. Smelling salts can be used to arouse patients to consciousness.

INTRAOPERATIVE PERIOD

Risks to Mohs Surgeons and Staff

While the majority of complications reviewed so far pertain to patients, there are risks to physicians and assistants as well. Acute injuries such as needlesticks and exposure to bloodborne pathogens can occur, as can more chronic injuries, including musculoskeletal complaints and carpal tunnel syndrome. It is important to mitigate these risks.

Maintaining an orderly surgical tray aids in safety and efficiency. Sharps, including scalpel blades, syringes with needles, and skin hooks, should be handled and stored with care. Suture needles have a tendency to "hitchhike" onto instruments, gauze, and gloves. Use of small, brightly colored pieces of foam has been reported to be an inexpensive and simple way to organize small sharps on the Mohs tray.[19] Other options for sharps storage on the Mohs tray include reusable medicine cups (metal, plastic, or glass), magnets, and commercially available surgical tray organizers.[19,20]

Universal precautions should be employed, including personal protective equipment, such as gloves, surgical masks, and face shields or goggles.[21] All medical personnel should be up to date on their vaccinations, including hepatitis B. Extra precautions, such as the use of gowns, double gloves, "no-touch" instrumentation techniques for reloading needle drivers, and blunt skin hooks can enhance the safety of the Mohs team, especially when operating on patients with known hepatitis C or HIV.[22] Nursing, histology, and cleaning staff should be made aware of the special needs of these patients so as to protect their privacy while maintaining the safety of staff and other patients. For known infectious patients, the authors dedicate a room on the day of surgery, keep all instruments in the room, and clean the room thoroughly after the procedure is completed and before using it for other patients. Postexposure prophylaxis protocols and employee health measures should be in place, and all members of the Mohs team should be aware of these plans. Another concern is the potential occupational risk of the smoke plume generated by electrosurgical devices, which will be discussed in the "Bleeding" section.

Ergonomics are an important and often overlooked aspect of Mohs surgery. Studies of Mohs surgeons indicate that musculoskeletal complaints, such as pain and stiffness of the neck, shoulders, and lower back, as well as headaches, are common and may begin early in a physician's career.[23] Despite the high prevalence of such complaints, many surgeons do not use ergonomic modifications in their practice.[24] One should consider ergonomics in all aspects of a Mohs day: performing surgery, reading slides at the microscope, and working at a desk or computer workstation. Proper patient and lighting position, whether the surgeon is seated or standing, is important for facilitating safe and effective surgery. For microscopes that are shared, there is an option that allows variable positioning of the main eyepieces to accommodate surgeons of various heights and desired head and eye positioning. Supportive footwear and comfortable flooring can help prevent musculoskeletal strain.[23] Ergonomic workstations with wrist rests for the keyboard and mouse, as well as lumbar support and footrests, are beneficial. The junior author has found considerable improvement from back strain and fatigue with the use of surgical loupes, which help maintain a comfortable working posture, as well as with daily stretches recommended by a physical therapist. These stretches utilize a high-density foam roller or bolster, which extends the spine and musculature to counteract the predominant daily working posture of flexion. Good nutrition and hydration are also important. The surgeon must remember to take care of him- or herself to ensure many years of successful practice and patient care.

Patient and Surgical Tray Errors

Since Mohs surgery is performed in stages, many surgeons have patients stay in a waiting room while their tissue is being processed and examined. This process improves efficiency, but it also carries some risks. Potential complications include bringing the wrong patient into a procedure room and using the wrong Mohs instrument tray. Some surgeons allow patients or their trays to stay in one room, but if the patient moves in and out, the correct patient still needs to be verified. Another approach, which can add to expense and staff labor, is to use a fresh set of instruments for each stage and subsequent reconstruction.

Consistent confirmation of correct patient and site by all involved staff prior to each Mohs stage and repair is paramount; this cannot be emphasized strongly enough. Systems and procedures that include double and triple checks, as discussed in the "Time-Outs and Checklists" section, should be in place to decrease errors. The Mohs surgeon should serve as a model of detail orientation, which should be observed and implemented by all staff. The senior author has found in his 20 years of practice that being detail–oriented is often a character trait that is either present or absent and cannot be taught to or learned by all staff. Early identification of those staff members who are not capable of this performance standard is critical, and removing them from the Mohs environment is imperative for patient safety and risk management. Such staff members may be easily distracted and often do not utilize checklists or other tools or procedures consistently.

Specimen and Laboratory Errors

Successful, safe, and efficient Mohs surgery involves teamwork and collaboration among the Mohs surgeon, surgical assistants, and histotechnicians. Careful tissue excision, orientation, handling, and verification are crucial. The Mohs surgeon starts the process by excising the tumor with precise beveling and marking of the peripheral margins with surgical hatches. The surgical hatches should be visible on both the excised tissue and the defect to enable accurate inking and grossing, as well as accurate mapping and treatment if positive margins are found. The hatches on the patient should not be so large as to interfere with cosmesis once tumor removal is complete; some surgeons use ink instead, such as gentian violet.

Communication between the Mohs surgeon and the histology technician is very important to ensure proper processing. The authors often have the technicians join them in the procedure room while stages are being taken to observe how the tissue is obtained, marked, and oriented. The technician can also draw a diagram of the tissue on the Mohs worksheet while the surgeon operates and then take the tissue to the laboratory once it has been removed to begin processing. Accurate diagramming of tissue specimen and hatch location is important, and the authors draw local anatomic landmarks (i.e., the eye, nose, or mouth) on the Mohs map in relation to the surgical site to help with orientation.

Tissue specimens should be clearly labeled with patient identifiers and handled carefully to maintain orientation and to avoid specimen mix-up. A technique utilizing a differently colored embedding medium for each individual patient has been proposed to help histology technicians avoid errors while processing multiple cases. In addition, using differently colored slide labels—which can be coordinated with the color of the embedding medium—can help Mohs surgeons easily identify the slides for a specific patient.[25] Systems to reduce specimen errors are important, particularly in high-volume Mohs practices, in which multiple surgeons are treating numerous patients on the same day. The authors prefer to treat one tumor on a patient at a time; however, if multiple tumors are treated with Mohs on the same patient in 1 day, techniques for differentiating the tissue specimens are also helpful to minimize error (Figure 4.2).

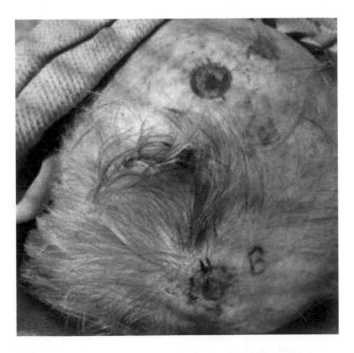

FIGURE 4.2   Two squamous cell carcinomas treated with Mohs surgery on the same day. The photo shows three surgical hatches at 12 o'clock on site A and two planned hatches at 12 o'clock on site B to differentiate tissue specimens.

Finally, proper storage and handling of chemicals in the Mohs lab, including ventilated hoods as necessitated by the chemicals being used, are required for staff and patient safety. In the United States, these are regulated by the Clinical Laboratory Improvement Amendments (CLIA) or the College of American Pathologists (CAP). Information on chemical storage and handling is included in the Material Safety Data Sheets (MSDSs), which should be stored in the laboratory upon receipt.

Bleeding

Intraoperative bleeding can be expected to occur during most Mohs cases. As discussed in Chapter 1, this may be further compounded by anticoagulant and antiplatelet medications, either prescribed or over-the-counter. Bleeding can obscure the surgical field if not adequately controlled. In addition, patients may experience postoperative bleeding and hematoma formation, which will be discussed in the "Hematoma, Seroma, and Ecchymoses" section. Detailed anatomical knowledge and preparation with electrosurgical units for hemostasis are a must for safe Mohs surgery.

As discussed earlier, epinephrine in the local anesthetic aids with intraoperative hemostasis and should be given time to allow maximum vasoconstriction. Bleeding is usually minor and easily controlled but can be significant, especially when arterial vessels are traumatized.

Mohs defects with minimal bleeding may be treated with cotton–tipped applicators or gauze soaked with aluminum chloride; the authors often utilize this technique for shallow nasal defects. Other useful materials for hemostasis, especially once the tumor has been removed and no further histological analysis is needed, include gelatin sponges (Gelfoam°, Pfizer Inc., New York, NY), cellulose products (Surgicel°, Ethicon Inc, Somerville, NJ), topical thrombin, microfibrillar collagen (Instat°, Ethicon Inc., Somerville, NJ), and kaolin impregnated gauze (QuikClot°, Z-Medica, Wallingford, CT). Less commonly used topical hemostatic agents are silver nitrate sticks and ferric subsulfate (i.e., Monsel solution); the latter is not recommended for Mohs, as it can cause hyperpigmentation, iatrogenic tattooing, and unusual reactive histology.[26]

Small bleeding veins, arterioles, and punctate dermal vessels can be controlled with electrodesiccation, electrofulguration, or electrocoagulation, as described in Chapter 2. Reviews of electrosurgical devices in patients with pacemakers and defibrillators indicate that their use is safe, and a recent *in vitro* study found hyfrecators to be safe for use in patients with defibrillators as well as pacemakers.[27] Patient safety has continued despite Mohs surgeons' moving away from previously recommended precautions, such as continuous intraoperative electrocardiographic monitoring for patients with pacemakers and magnetic inactivation of defibrillators with cardiologist approval.[28] Battery powered electrocautery devices can also be used for hemostasis and pose no risk for patients with implantable electronic devices, since they deliver heat rather than electrical energy. In addition to cardiac devices, patients may have electronic nerve stimulators and other implantable devices.

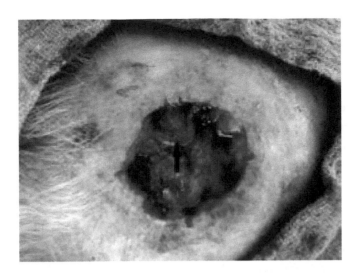

FIGURE 4.3   Intact superficial temporal artery in the base of a Mohs defect on the right forehead.

Another consideration with electrosurgical devices is the growing body of evidence that indicates the vapor or smoke plume generated not only is irritating to the respiratory tract but also may contain infectious particles (particularly human papilloma virus) and has *in vitro* mutagenic potential. Standard surgical masks alone do not provide adequate protection against this occupational hazard; however, smoke evacuators or filters offer additional safety for the surgeon, staff, and patient.[29,30,31] The United States Department of Labor's Occupational Safety and Health Administration (OSHA) recognizes the potential risks of surgical smoke plumes but does not currently have specific standards for regulation or prophylaxis against their hazards.[32] The authors find that biterminal forceps emit less of a smoke plume than monoterminal devices.

When transected, larger vessels require suture ligation at both ends with a figure-of-eight technique. Hemostats are useful for clamping larger bleeding vessels prior to ligation. Extra care should be taken when operating on the temple, as the superficial temporal artery and its branches may be encountered and can cause significant bleeding challenges (Figure 4.3). Occasionally, surgical drains may be needed for large wounds with significant bleeding. Rarely, arterial bleeding cannot be controlled in the Mohs suite and patients must be managed in a more controlled operating room setting, where they may even require blood products or reversal of anticoagulation.[33] It is imperative to have protocols in place for such emergencies.

Horizontal mattress or running locked sutures, direct manual pressure, and pressure dressings are additional useful hemostatic techniques, as noted in Chapter 2. Patients should be instructed to limit their activity and to refrain from heavy lifting and exercise postoperatively. Ice may also be used to decrease postoperative bleeding by vasoconstriction.[34]

Nerve Trauma

Sensory and motor nerves may be damaged during Mohs surgery. Nerve deficits may also result postoperatively with scar tissue and fibrosis entrapping small nerves. Preoperative nerve deficits should be identified and documented prior to anesthesia. Motor nerve function should be evaluated before and after each operative stage, as local anesthetics can cause temporary paralysis. Patients should be reassured that this effect resolves once the anesthetic has worn off. Surgeons must be familiar with anatomic danger zones and discuss risks with patients whose tumors are located in such regions (Figure 4.4).

Motor nerve deficits are the most significant nerve complications from Mohs surgery. Paralysis is permanent loss of motor nerve function and usually results from complete transection of a nerve, whereas paresis is defined as slight or partial paralysis. Neuropraxia is a temporary conduction deficit caused by trauma or stretching of a nerve.[35]

The facial nerve (seventh cranial nerve, or CN VII) is the main motor nerve of the face and has five major branches: temporal, zygomatic, buccal, marginal mandibular, and cervical. The extratemporal trunk of the facial nerve, which gives rise to these branches, is rarely encountered during Mohs surgery. This is due to its deep location, inferior to the tragus, where it crosses the styloid process to enter the deep tissue of the parotid gland (Figure 4.5). The temporal (also known as the frontal) branch of CN VII is the motor nerve most commonly injured in facial surgery, given its superficial location over the temporal fascia just below the superficial muscular aponeurotic system (SMAS) as it crosses the zygomatic arch.[35] This danger zone, known as Pitanguy's line in the plastic surgical literature, encompasses a line from the tragus to the lateral eyebrow (Figure 4.6).

The temporal nerve has multiple branches, and deficits depend on where the injury occurs; a proximal injury results in greater loss of function than a more distal trauma. Proximal

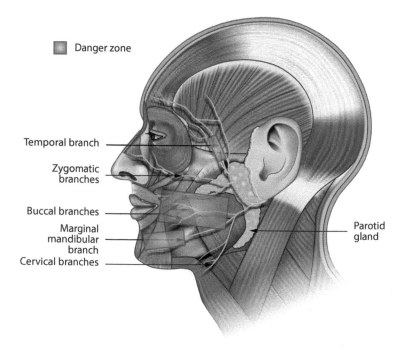

FIGURE 4.4   Diagram of motor nerve danger zones of the head and neck.

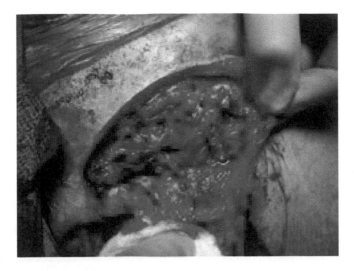

FIGURE 4.5   Right facial nerve trunk in the parotid gland exposed during superficial parotidectomy for deeply invasive squamous cell carcinoma. (Photo courtesy of Ron Walker, M.D., assistant professor, Head and Neck Oncology, Microvascular Reconstruction, Saint Louis University.)

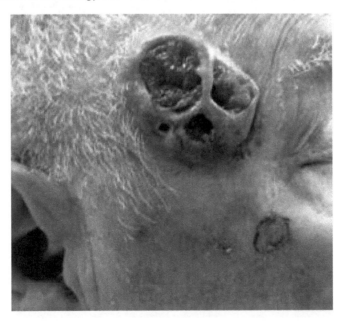

FIGURE 4.6   Large squamous cell carcinoma overlying the right frontal branch danger zone.

transection of the temporal nerve may result in unilateral forehead paralysis with resultant brow ptosis. Ptosis can be exacerbated by resection of the frontalis muscle in cases of deeply invasive tumors (Figures 4.7 and 4.8). There is the potential for reinnervation, especially for more distal defects. If a nerve is transected intraoperatively and the severed ends are visible, reanastomosis with a thin suture, such as 6-0 polyglactin 910 (Vicryl, Ethicon Inc., Somerville, NJ), can be attempted. The patient may also be referred to colleagues in head and

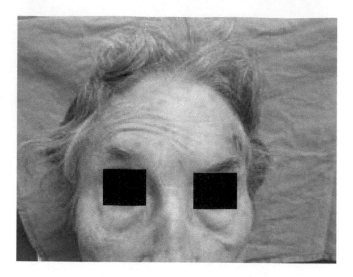

FIGURE 4.7   Left frontal branch paralysis after Mohs surgery for left temple recurrent, infiltrative basal cell carcinoma.

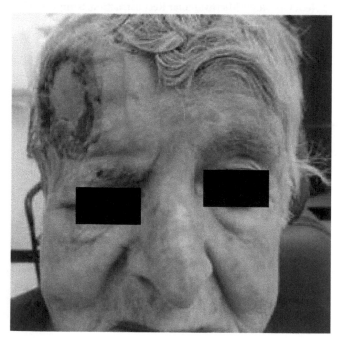

FIGURE 4.8   Marked right brow/eyelid ptosis after Mohs excision to bone for deeply invasive, recurrent squamous cell carcinoma. The patient's treatment was complicated by right frontal branch nerve and superior temporal artery transection; significant edema is contributing to the ptosis.

neck or plastic surgery, who may have more experience managing facial nerve injury, both acutely and in the long term.

The marginal mandibular branch of CN VII (Figure 4.4) is another superficial motor nerve susceptible to trauma during Mohs surgery, and injury can result in an asymmetric smile. Damage to the spinal accessory nerve (11th cranial nerve, or CN XI) can occur with surgery in Erb's point and results in winging of the scapula, as well as shoulder and neck weakness.

Sensory deficits, such as paresthesias, may result from damage to small, unnamed cutaneous nerves, but these usually resolve with time and do not result in significant problems for patients. Neuropathic pain can, in rare cases, result from sensory nerve damage.[34] Damage to larger, named sensory nerves can occur during Mohs; the more common deficits include persistent scalp numbness from damage to the supraorbital or supratrochlear nerve. Earlobe numbness may result from trauma to the greater auricular nerve, which may be encountered with deep resections of the upper neck, below the earlobe and above the level of the sternocleidomastoid muscle (Figures 4.9 and 4.10).

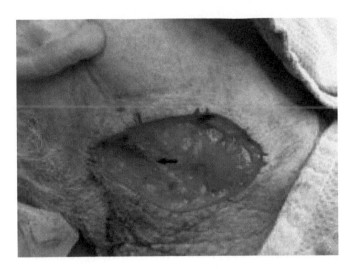

FIGURE 4.9   Right greater auricular nerve overlying the sternocleidomastoid muscle in the base of a Mohs defect.

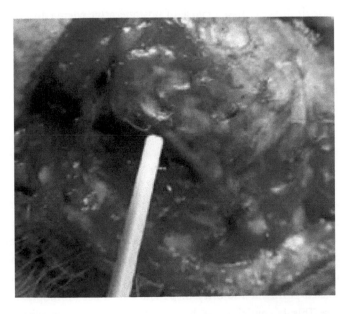

FIGURE 4.10   The right greater auricular nerve was inadvertently transected during extirpation of a squamous cell carcinoma. Three 6-0 Vicryl sutures were used to reapproximate the nerve. The patient had postoperative right earlobe numbness, which has subsequently resolved.

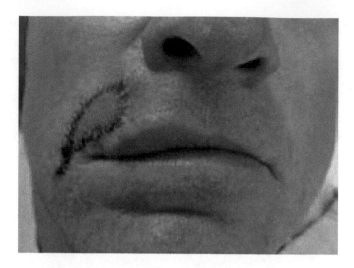

FIGURE 4.11   Right mucosal lip edema immediately after Mohs and V-Y flap for right upper cutaneous lip basal cell carcinoma.

Edema

Edema, or soft tissue swelling, can occur intraoperatively and postoperatively. Causes include tissue trauma and infiltration of local anesthetic. Nerve blocks can help reduce the local tissue edema associated with ring blocks but do not offer the vasoconstrictive advantage of epinephrine. Edema can be expected to resolve with time but can lead to intraoperative reconstructive challenges, particularly when determining how much tissue needs to be excised for standing cones ("dog-ears").

Impaired lymphatic drainage is also a cause of postoperative edema and commonly occurs with lower eyelid and medial cheek repairs. Overall, the mucosal lip (Figure 4.11) and the eyelids are the two most common sites that tend to become quite edematous during Mohs surgery. The nasal mucosa may also become edematous after nasal surgery and reconstruction, but this can be expected to improve with time and scar massage, so long as the external nasal valve is competent.

POSTOPERATIVE PERIOD
Pain

Pain after Mohs surgery usually is mild and resolves within a few days. A prospective study found the highest pain scores were associated with the day of surgery, when 52% of patients took analgesics, with a steady decline by postoperative day 4, with only 5% of patients using analgesics at that time.[36] This study also found that flap and graft repairs caused more pain than linear closures and second intent healing and that younger age (<66 years old) was associated with increased pain. The majority of patients used acetaminophen, with only 7.1% needing narcotics. This is consistent with the authors' practice, in which patients rarely require analgesics stronger than acetaminophen for postoperative analgesia. Significant or worsening pain may be a symptom of wound infection, hematoma, or other postoperative complication and warrants a follow-up examination.

The ear is a unique site that may become painful due to chondritis, either infectious or inflammatory, particularly when cartilage is traumatized. Nonsteroidal anti-inflammatory drugs (NSAIDs) may alleviate the pain of chondritis, but infection should be ruled out, as the ear is often colonized by the Gram-negative bacterium *Pseudomonas aeruginosa* (Figure 4.12). Fluoroquinolones, such as ciprofloxacin or levofloxacin, are typically used for *Pseudomonas* infections. Although a more detailed discussion of potential medication side effects is outside the scope of this chapter, it should be noted that fluoroquinolones pose a risk for tendonitis or tendon rupture and have an FDA black box warning stating that this risk is increased in patients more than 60 years old; patients on corticosteroids; and patients with kidney, heart, or lung transplants.

A study of Mohs reconstructions involving auricular cartilage found complications to be rare when appropriate surgical technique and perioperative anti-pseudomonal antibiotics were administered.[37] The need for prophylactic antibiotics for ear surgery is unclear, as another study found no post-Mohs wound infections at this site without the use of antibiotics.[38] Studies of second intent healing of auricular surgical sites have demonstrated that the routine prophylactic use of oral or topical antibiotics does not confer advantages over regular local wound care.[39,40]

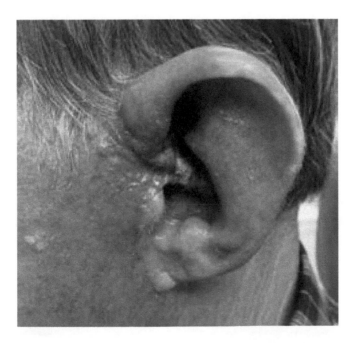

FIGURE 4.12 Culture confirmed *Pseudomonas aeruginosa* infection of left preauricular cheek/ helical root defect repaired with complex closure with Burow's graft. The infection resolved with oral ciprofloxacin and silver sulfadiazine cream.

Infection

The overall reported surgical site infection (SSI) rates for dermatological surgery range from 0.07% to 4.25%.[41] Even though Mohs wounds are classified as non-sterile or clean contaminated, studies have shown exceedingly low risk for infections. A well-designed prospective study that excluded patients on antibiotics found an SSI rate of 0.91% when using clean technique and clean gloves with one sterile instrument pack for the entire Mohs case including reconstruction.[41] There does appear to be a slightly increased risk for SSI when performing flap reconstructions .[38,41,42] While some studies have found increased SSI rates with grafts and surgery below the knee,[42] others have not.[38,41]

The most common SSIs are bacterial. Postoperative bacterial wound infections are characterized by pain, erythema, purulent discharge, honey-colored crusting, and malodor; occasionally, patients may become febrile (Figure 4.13). The majority of infections are caused by methicillin-sensitive *Staphylococcus aureus* (MSSA), although the incidence of methicillin-resistant *S. aureus* (MRSA) infections is increasing. Other Gram-positive bacteria, such as group A *Streptococcus,* can also cause wound infections and are more commonly associated with symptoms of infectious lymphangitis and more rapid onset of symptoms. Gram-negative wound infections occur with lower frequency, although certain sites, such as the ear, are at higher risk, as discussed in the section "Pain." Abscesses are uncommon; they should be drained, irrigated with sterile saline, and packed with iodoform gauze. Warm compresses, as well as antibiotics, can aid in the resolution of abscesses.

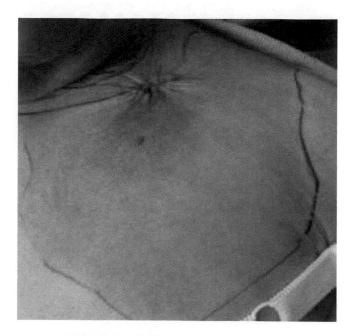

FIGURE 4.13   Methicillin-sensitive *Staphylococcus aureus* (MSSA) cellulitis complicating a purse string closure of a left clavicle graft donor site. This was treated with oral doxycycline and silver sulfadiazine cream.

In our practice, suspected wound infections are cultured to confirm infection and to identify the pathogenic bacteria and their sensitivity. We commonly prescribe topical antibiotics for suspected SSIs, with our preference being silver sulfadiazine cream for its broad antibacterial coverage (both Gram-positive and Gram-negative bacteria, including MRSA and *Pseudomonas*). Topical silver sulfadiazine has a theoretical risk for contact sensitization in patients with sulfonamide allergy and can rarely cause brown-gray hyperpigmentation.[43] Mupirocin provides good Gram-positive coverage, including MRSA, and sensitization is uncommon. A relatively new topical antibiotic ointment, retapamulin, also has Gram-positive coverage, but it is not indicated for MRSA. Over-the-counter antibiotics, such as bacitracin and triple antibiotic ointment (bacitracin/neomycin/polymyxin B) may be used, but caution should be exercised, as bacitracin and neomycin are common causes of allergic contact dermatitis, especially in patients with stasis dermatitis.[43] Topical gentamicin and polymyxin B have good Gram-negative coverage, including for *Pseudomonas*.

Oral antibiotics may be needed for confirmed bacterial infection, with first- and second-generation cephalosporins (i.e., cephalexin) often used for MSSA infections. In cases of MRSA infections, doxycycline, trimethoprim-sulfamethoxazole, or clindamycin may be used. Proper use and side effects of all prescribed medications should be thoroughly discussed with patients.

Herpes simplex virus (HSV) wound infections have been reported to occur rarely after dermatologic surgery, though care should be taken in patients who have active herpetic outbreaks.[44] The senior author has managed cases of very subtle HSV wound infections presenting with only a focal erosion, crust, or vesicle, but with complaints of pain out of proportion to clinical exam findings. Candidal infections can also occur rarely, especially in moist, occluded sites, such as the groin or axilla.[34]

Hematoma, Seroma, and Ecchymoses

Hematomas can impair wound healing, cause epidermal necrosis, and serve as a nidus of infection.[34] An acute hematoma should be suspected when a patient complains of increasing pain and swelling at the surgical site. Thick "black currant jelly" discharge is a sign of a coagulated, organized hematoma. Hematomas with active bleeding require opening of the wound and hemostasis. Acute hematomas that are not actively bleeding should be evacuated with a large-bore needle and syringe (Figures 4.14 and 4.15). On the other hand, the thick coagulum of a stable and organizing hematoma requires evacuation after sutures are removed or observation if it is small and improving. If hematomas are opened, they should be irrigated and packed with iodoform gauze.[34] The authors perform bacterial cultures of hematoma contents and treat with empiric antibiotics, given the increased risk for infection.

Seromas are serous fluid collections that can clinically mimic hematomas. Layered closures that eliminate dead space decrease the risk for seroma. Seromas can be drained in a manner similar to that used for hematoma, with a large-bore needle on a syringe. If the discharge is cloudy or purulent, bacterial culture should be performed and antibiotics started.[34]

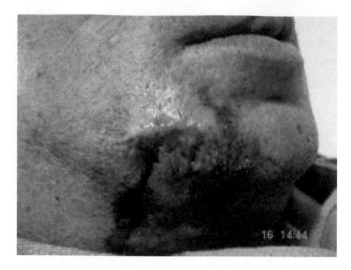

FIGURE 4.14   Acute draining hematoma on the right chin after Mohs surgery and repair.

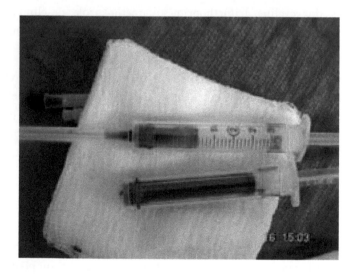

FIGURE 4.15   Blood drained from hematoma.

Ecchymoses may be quite prominent, particularly with surgery above or around the eyes (Figure 4.16). Patients should be counseled as to the self-limited nature of bruising and advised to use ice. Gravity may result in ecchymoses developing quite a distance below the surgical site, and patient education is helpful when this is anticipated.

Dermatitis and Suture Reactions

Inflammatory conditions, such dermatitis and suture reactions, may clinically mimic infection. Suture granulomas may form with the use of buried absorbable suture and may appear as papules or nodules along the suture line (Figure 4.17). These can be expected to resolve with time, but occasionally the offending stitch may be eliminated through the

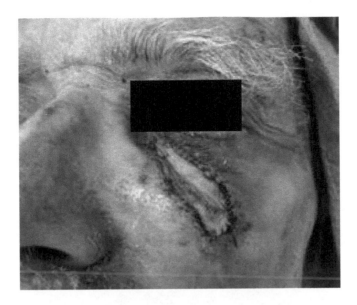

FIGURE 4.16   Left periorbital ecchymosis after Mohs surgery and graft repair.

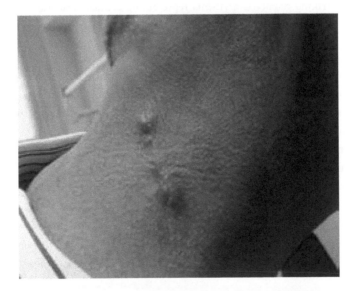

FIGURE 4.17   Suture granulomas at the poles of a right neck primary closure, which used a buried absorbable subcuticular suture technique. Light growth of MRSA was cultured from the wound, and the papules resolved over time with oral doxycycline.

skin. These "spitting" sutures may present as an intact suture or as a more digested, sterile, inflammatory pustule; the former can be removed with suture scissors, while the latter is easily incised and drained. The possibility of spitting sutures should be discussed with the patient to alleviate concerns should this occur. In the senior author's experience, spitting sutures usually occur approximately 6–8 weeks postoperatively, which is a good time to see a patient for follow-up.

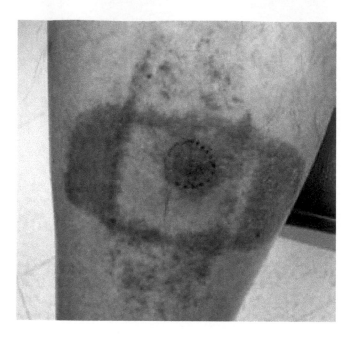

FIGURE 4.18   Striking geometric erythema representing contact dermatitis reaction to bandage adhesive on leg.

Adhesive on wound dressings and antibiotic or healing ointments may cause either an irritant or an allergic contact dermatitis. Geometric erythema in the distribution of the bandage or the site of the ointment application is a clue to contact dermatitis, as is pruritus (Figure 4.18). Bacterial cultures may be performed if infection cannot be ruled out. As discussed earlier, bacitracin and neomycin can cause allergic contact dermatitis. In addition, a recent study found increased wound erythema with Aquaphor Healing Ointment' (Beiersdorf AG, Hamburg, Germany), which contains the potential allergens lanolin and bisabolol, compared to plain white petrolatum.[45] Thus, the authors recommend petroleum ointment squeezed from a tube (rather than applied from a jar, to decrease the risk of contamination) for routine postoperative wound care. Treatment of contact dermatitis involves discontinuation of the offending agent and the use of a topical corticosteroid for more severe cases.

Dehiscence, Epidermolysis, and Necrosis

Dehiscence is the opening of a sutured wound. and usually results from wound tension, poor surgical technique, premature suture removal, or pressure from hematoma, abscess, or seroma (Figure 4.19). Epidermolysis is the superficial shedding or crusting of the epidermis overlying a repair and is usually the result of impaired circulation. Necrosis occurs with tissue infarction from vascular compromise and manifests as a black eschar over the reconstruction, usually a flap or graft (Figures 4.20a and b). Risk factors for necrosis include tension, a small, inadequate, or compromised flap pedicle, crush injury to grafts, infection, hematoma, and seroma. As discussed in Chapter 1, tobacco smokers are at

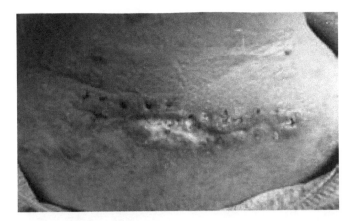

FIGURE 4.19   Dehiscence of a posterior neck closure complicated by culture-proven MRSA infection, which resolved with doxycycline and silver sulfadiazine cream.

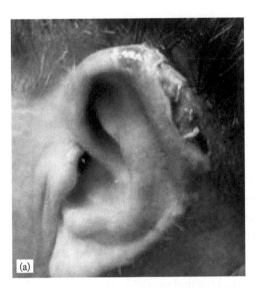
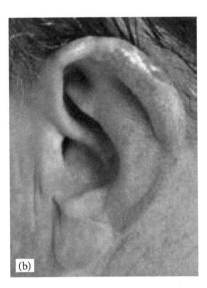

FIGURE 4.20   (a) Partial left postauricular interpolation flap necrosis in a patient with *Klebsiella oxytoca* infection. Infection was treated with oral ciprofloxacin and silver sulfadiazine cream (b) Left postauricular interpolation flap 3 months postoperatively. The wound is nearly fully healed, with good cosmesis..

increased risk for wound dehiscence, flap or graft necrosis, prolonged healing, and infections (Figure 4.21).[46] Patients with diabetes mellitus are also reported to be at increased risk for graft failure.[47]

These complications are typically managed conservatively with petrolatum and bandages to allow healing by second intent; infarcted flaps and grafts are usually left in place to serve as biological dressings. Epidermolysis typically resolves with minimal cosmetic repercussions. Dehiscence and necrosis can lead to more prominent scars, but the final result is often much better than what is anticipated early in the postoperative period (Figure 4.20a and b).

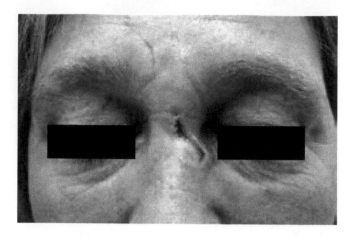

FIGURE 4.21   Partial glabella transposition flap necrosis in a heavy smoker.

Maintaining close and frequent follow-ups reassures patients that the surgeon is committed to helping them attain the best possible outcome.

Abnormal Scarring

Any cutaneous surgical procedure, including Mohs surgery, that extends to the depth of the dermis may result in a scar. As discussed in Chapters 2 and 3, careful surgical technique, positioning of scars in rhytides and in junctions of cosmetic subunits, and the use of optimal reconstructive methods aid in achieving the best aesthetic outcomes. It should be noted that different patients often have very different expectations and ideals: some may prefer limited reconstruction and not mind more prominent scarring, while others demand the highest of cosmetic outcomes. The authors advise their Mohs patients that scars are unavoidable but that they will attempt to make them as minimally noticeable as possible.

Counseling patients on typical expectations and normal wound healing and remodeling is important. Everted edges of the wound may be somewhat perplexing to a patient expecting a flat scar when removing the dressing for the first time; the rationale for and the expected results from such eversion should therefore be explained. Fresh scars are often erythematous and should fade with time, sometimes with resultant hypopigmentation (Figure 4.22).

Unfortunately, no matter how skilled the surgeon, results may sometimes be less than ideal. As discussed in Chapter 5, certain patients, such as patients with darker skin, may be more prone to developing hypertrophic or keloidal scars. In addition, patients with skin of color often heal with postoperative hyperpigmentation (Figure 4.23). Flaps and grafts may heal with a bulky appearance, known as a trapdoor defect or pincushioning (Figure 4.24). Spread or "fish-mouth" scars are often encountered at anatomic sites under considerable tension, such as the chest and back (Figure 4.25). "Train track" scars result from epidermal sutures that are placed under too much tension or left in place for too long.

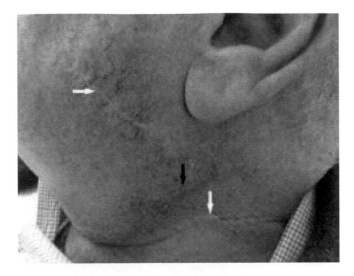

FIGURE 4.22   Fresh, pink everted scar on the right jawline (black arrow), in contrast with healed hypopigmented scars (white arrows).

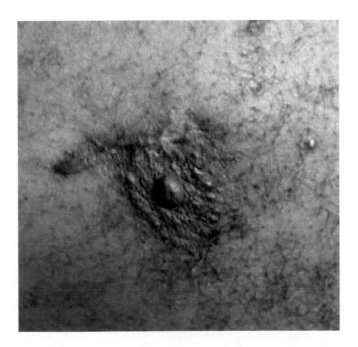

FIGURE 4.23   Hyperpigmented hypertrophic scar on the chest of a patient with dark skin.

Aside from being cosmetically displeasing, scars may also cause functional impairment, constrictive scar bands over a joint, or scars causing ectropion or eclabium, as detailed in the section "Distortion of Free Margins and Site-Specific Considerations." It should also be kept in mind that it is socially acceptable for women to wear makeup and potentially camouflage scars or dyspigmentation, while this is not usually the case with men.

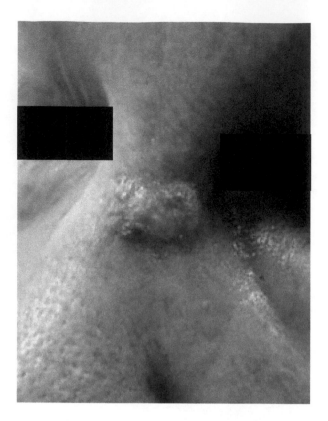

FIGURE 4.24 Hypertrophic ("pincushioned") full-thickness skin graft on the nasal dorsum 1 month postoperatively.

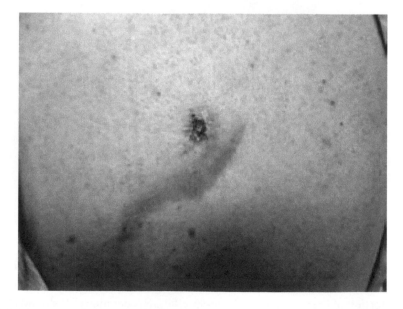

FIGURE 4.25 A spread scar on the back of a patient. There is also a recent biopsy scar superiorly.

While surgical techniques discussed in Chapters 2 and 3 help to reduce the risk of abnormal healing, various procedures in the postoperative period may be employed to correct objectionable scarring. These will be addressed in Part II of this book.

Distortion of Free Margins and Site-Specific Considerations

Free margins may become distorted as a consequence of improper tension resulting from repairs or from the contraction of second intent wound healing. Pulling or distortion of free margins may cause issues not only with cosmesis but also with functional impairment.

The eyelids are susceptible to ectropion (eversion, or turning out), which, in severe cases, can cause difficulty closing the lids and can result in dry eye and corneal irritation (Figure 4.26). The lower lid is most commonly affected by ectropion; its ability to resist tension can be checked preoperatively with the snap or tug test. In the process, the lid is retracted downward from the globe and released. A return to initial position within 1-2 seconds without blinking indicates a normal snap test.[20] During and after eyelid, cheek, or temple repairs, tension on the lower eyelid can be checked by having the patient sit upright or semi-reclined and gaze upward while opening the mouth fully (Figure 4.27).[48] In addition, surgery on the medial

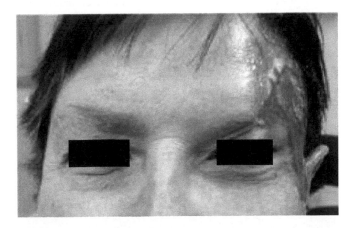

FIGURE 4.26   Left lateral ectropion secondary to contraction during a multi-staged excision for a large, recurrent basal cell carcinoma. The patient had oculoplastic repair once the tumor was removed.

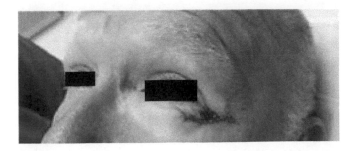

FIGURE 4.27   Patient with mouth agape and an upward gaze, demonstrating lack of tension on the left lower eyelid after primary closure.

canthus can traumatize the lacrimal canalicular system, which would require oculoplastic reconstruction. Eyebrow position must also be respected, as unilateral upward pull can cause a quizzical look.

Eclabium is eversion of the lip, which is not cosmetically pleasing and, in severe cases, can cause problems with creating a tight oral seal (Figure 4.28). In addition, notching of the vermilion border can occur following lip repair and is often quite problematic to the patient. As discussed in Chapter 3, edema and vasoconstriction from anesthetic can blanch the pink of the mucosal lip, making this important cosmetic junction difficult to appreciate during surgery. Preoperative marking with a surgical pen or gentian violet ink helps with proper alignment in such repairs.

The auricular helix may become crumpled, cupped, or bowed when structural support is lost with the removal of cartilage (Figure 4.29). Repair using a graft, a flap, or a wedge excision may help to reduce this complication.

Nasal alar rim notching is cosmetically unacceptable to most patients and can be a consequence of undue tension on the ala (Figure 4.30). In addition, nasal airflow can be significantly obstructed by the pinching effect of wound contraction following various surgical closures or by the collapse of the external nasal valve. The latter usually occurs secondary to the removal of supportive nasal tissue without appropriate fixation of the nasal valve.

Additional Considerations

Hair-bearing sites deserve special attention with Mohs surgery and reconstruction. As discussed in Chapter 3, alopecia may result when scalp surgery extends below the level of the follicles or with significant follicular trauma. In addition, alopecia secondary to surgery on the upper cutaneous lip, lateral cheeks, sideburn areas, and chin in male patients who wear beards or mustaches

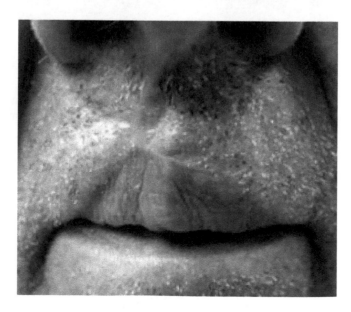

FIGURE 4.28   Right upper lip eclabium.

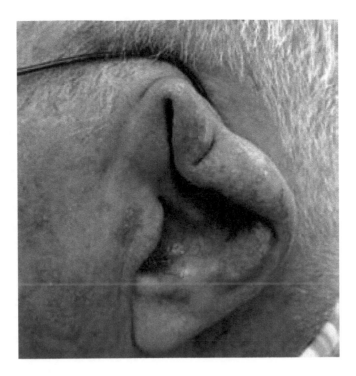

FIGURE 4.29   Crumpling of superior aspect of left helix after extensive Mohs surgery. The patient had refused repair and was pleased with the final result, as he was still able to wear glasses and had no functional impairment.

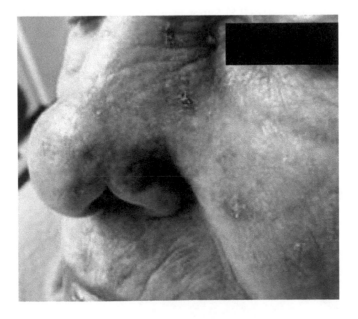

FIGURE 4.30   Left alar notch.

is also a concern. Conversely, unwanted hair can complicate full-thickness grafts that contain terminal hair follicles or scalp-to-ear interpolation flaps. Laser hair removal and electrolysis are options for epilation, but it is best to avoid such complications with proper donor site selection.

Deeply invasive tumors on sites such as the scalp, forehead, and temples may require removal of periosteum and exposure of the underlying bone. Mohs surgeons should be aware of the rare but serious complication of cerebral air embolism, which has been reported to occur during Mohs on the scalp with exposure of calvarium.[49] Exposure of bone may also result from infection of surgical sites or from desiccation of the overlying soft tissue when healing by granulation (Figure 4.31). Complex reconstructive techniques, such as flaps, grafts, or free flaps, may be needed for repair of such defects. The authors have had great success using bovine xenografts to heal exposed bone in patients who do not desire or cannot tolerate more involved reconstructions. The wounds are kept moist with petrolatum to encourage granulation, although healing may be prolonged. Occasionally, exposed bone, often desiccated and sometimes necrotic, persists, and other measures, such as curetting or chiseling of the outer bony cortex to stimulate small bleeding points and to promote granulation, are needed. Allowing wounds to heal by second intent or with xenografts may result in "proud flesh," or hypergranulation, which can be treated with acetic acid soaks or silver nitrate sticks.[20]

Life-Threatening Complications

Fortunately, life-threatening complications are rare in Mohs surgery. Myocardial infarction, cardiopulmonary arrest, and cerebrovascular events may occur and require immediate activation of the EMS. Mohs surgeons and staff should be trained in basic life support (BLS) or advanced cardiac life support (ACLS). Supplemental oxygen and automated external defibrillators (AEDs) may be kept in the office for use in such emergencies.

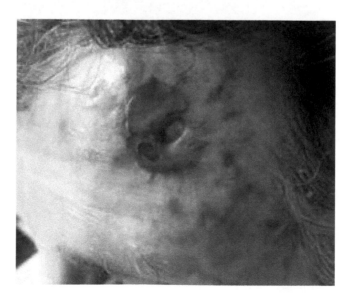

FIGURE 4.31   Granulating left forehead wound with a small central focus of necrosis down to bone, requiring prolonged healing.

Anaphylaxis can occur and can quickly progress to airway obstruction. Epinephrine autoinjectors (EpiPen, Mylan Specialty L.P., Basking Ridge, NJ) may provide immediate treatment for this life-threatening type I hypersensitivity reaction. As discussed in the section "Reactions to Antiseptics and Anesthetics," severe lidocaine toxicity can also be life-threatening.

The authors have had one patient who experienced a postoperative pulmonary embolism secondary to deep vein thrombosis (DVT), likely present preoperatively, after surgery on the affected leg; additionally, there is a report of post-Mohs DVT in the literature.[50] Finally, one of the author's patients developed a large and rapidly expanding hematoma two days after surgery on the neck, which required intubation in order to secure and protect the airway.

CONCLUSIONS

Complications can occur with any medical treatment, including Mohs surgery. Managing complications in a timely manner while addressing patient concerns and anxiety results in the best possible outcomes. Staff members who answer and triage patient phone calls should be knowledgeable about potential postoperative complications and be able to recognize when patients require immediate physician evaluation. Conveying care and a commitment to the ultimate outcome goes a long way in working through the uncomfortable experience of any complication.

Finally, it is important to learn from personal experience as well as the experience of others. Some cases or complications may require management beyond our own level of training and expertise. It is essential to know one's own limitations and to recognize when to enlist the expertise of colleagues in other fields, such as emergency medicine, plastic surgery, otolaryngology, and oculoplastic surgery (Figure 4.32).

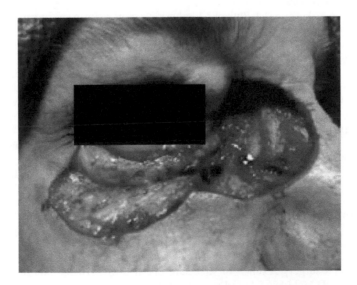

FIGURE 4.32   Large defect of the right lower eyelid, medial canthus, and nose after Mohs surgery for a basal cell carcinoma. The patient was referred to oculoplastic surgery for repair.

REFERENCES

1. Cook JL, Perone JB.A prospective evaluation of the incidence of complications associated with Mohs micrographic surgery. *Arch Dermatol* 2003;139(2):143–52.
2. Bordeaux JS, Martires KJ, Goldberg D, Pattee SF, Fu P, Maloney ME. Prospective evaluation of dermatologic surgery complications including patients on multiple antiplatelet and anticoagulant medications. *J Am Acad Dermatol* 2011;65(3):576–83.
3. Delaney A, Shimizu I, Goldberg LH, MacFarlane DF. Life expectancy after Mohs micrographic surgery in patients aged 90 years and older. *J Am Acad Dermatol* 2013;68(2):296–300.
4. Haynes AB, Weiser TG, Berry WR, et al. A surgical safety checklist to reduce morbidity and mortality in a global population. *N Engl J Med* 2009;360(5):491–9.
5. Borchard A, Schwappach DL, Barbir A, Bezzola P. A systematic review of the effectiveness, compliance, and critical factors for implementation of safety checklists in surgery. *Ann Surg* 2012;256(6):925–33.
6. Bliss LA, Ross-Richardson CB, Sanzari LJ, et al. Thirty-day outcomes support implementation of a surgical safety checklist. *J Am Coll Surg* 2012;215(6):766–76.
7. Weiser TG, Haynes AB, Lashoher A, et al. Perspectives in quality: Designing the WHO Surgical Safety Checklist. *Int J Qual Health Care* 2010;22(5):365–70.
8. World Alliance for Patient Safety. 2008. WHO surgical safety checklist and implementation manual. [online] Available at: http://www.who.int/patientsafety/safesurgery/ss_checklist/en/index.html [Accessed: 21 Jan 2014].
9. Levy SM, Senter CE, Hawkins RB, et al. Implementing a surgical checklist: More than checking a box. *Surgery* 2012;152(3):331–6.
10. Nemeth SA, Lawrence N. Site identification challenges in dermatologic surgery: A physician survey. *J Am Acad Dermatol* 2012;67(2):262–8.
11. Rossy KM, Lawrence N. Difficulty with surgical site identification: What role does it play in dermatology? *J Am Acad Dermatol* 2012;67(2):257–61.
12. McGinness JL, Goldstein G. The value of preoperative biopsy-site photography for identifying cutaneous lesions. *Dermatol Surg* 2010;36(2):194–7.
13. Ke M, Moul D, Camouse M, et al. Where is it? The utility of biopsy-site photography. *Dermatol Surg* 2010;36(2):198–202.
14. Chuang GS, Gilchrest BA. Ultraviolet-fluorescent tattoo location of cutaneous biopsy site. *Dermatol Surg* 2012;38(3):479–83.
15. Lee SK, Zhai H, Maibach HI. Allergic contact dermatitis from iodine preparations: A conundrum. *Contact Dermatitis* 2005;52(4):184–7.
16. Lai P, Coulson C, Pothier DD, Rutka J. Chlorhexidine ototoxicity in ear surgery, part 1: Review of the literature. *J Otolaryngol Head Neck Surg* 2011;40(6):437–40.
17. Huether M, Brodland D. Local anesthetics. In: Wolverton S (ed). *Comprehensive Dermatologic Drug Therapy,* 2nd ed. Philadelphia: Saunders Elsevier; 2007.
18. McKee DE, Lalonde DH, Thoma A, Glennie DL, Hayward JE. Optimal time delay between epinephrine injection and incision to minimize bleeding. *Plast Reconstr Surg* 2013;131(4):811–4.
19. Chrastil B, Wanitphakdeedecha R, Nguyen TH, Chen TM. A simple, inexpensive means to minimize suture "hitchhiker" sharps injury in the setting of a limited surgical workspace. *Dermatol Surg* 2008;34(9):1226–7.
20. Salasche SJ, Orengo IF, Siegle RJ. *Dermatologic Surgery Tips and Techniques.* Philadelphia: Mosby Elsevier; 2007, pp. 40, 108, 180.
21. Holzmann RD, Liang M, Nadiminti H, et al. Blood exposure risk during procedural dermatology. *J Am Acad Dermatol* 2008;58(5):817–25.
22. LoPiccolo MC, Balle MR, Kouba DJ. Safety precautions in Mohs micrographic surgery for patients with known blood-borne infections: A survey-based study. *Dermatol Surg* 2012;38(7 Pt 1):1059–65.
23. Esser AC, Koshy JG, Randle HW. Ergonomics in office-based surgery: A survey-guided observational study. *Dermatol Surg* 2007;33(11):1304–13.
24. Liang CA, Levine VJ, Dusza SW, Hale EK, Nehal KS. Musculoskeletal disorders and ergonomics in dermatologic surgery: A survey of Mohs surgeons in 2010. *Dermatol Surg* 2012;38(2):240–8.
25. Housewright CD, Goldstein GD. Color coordinating embedding medium and slide labels to reduce errors in Mohs surgery. *Dermatol Surg* 2012;38(7 Pt 1):1071–2.

26. Forman SB. Miscellaneous topical agents. In: Wolverton S (ed). *Comprehensive Dermatologic Drug Therapy.* 2nd ed. Philadelphia: Saunders Elsevier; 2007, p 779.

27. Weyer C, Siegle RJ, Eng GG. Investigation of hyfrecators and their in vitro interference with implantable cardiac devices. *Dermatol Surg* 2012;38(11):1843–8.

28. Riordan AT, Gamache C, Fosko SW. Electrosurgery and cardiac devices. *J Am Acad Dermatol* 1997;37(2 Pt 1):250–5.

29. Alp E, Bijl D, Bleichrodt RP, Hansson B, Voss A. Surgical smoke and infection control. *J Hosp Infect* 2006;62(1):1–5.

30. Hill DS, O'Neill JK, Powell RJ, Oliver DW. Surgical smoke—a health hazard in the operating theatre: A study to quantify exposure and a survey of the use of smoke extractor systems in UK plastic surgery units. *J Plast Reconstr Aesthet Surg* 2012;65(7):911–6.

31. Lewin JM, Brauer JA, Ostad A. Surgical smoke and the dermatologist. *J Am Acad Dermatol* 2011;65(3):636–41.

32. OSHA.gov. 2014. Laser/Electrosurgery Plume. https://www.osha.gov/SLTC/laserelectrosurgeryplume/index.html. Accessed January 21, 2014.

33. Hurst EA, Yu SS, Grekin RC, Neuhaus IM. Bleeding complications in dermatologic surgery. *Semin Cutan Med Surg* 2007;26(4):189–95.

34. Allen EJ, Youker RS. Surgical complications. In: Vidimos AT, Ammirati CT, Poblete-Lopez C (eds). *Dermatologic Surgery.* New York: Elsevier; 2009.

35. Hendi A. Temporal nerve neuropraxia and contralateral compensatory brow elevation. *Dermatol Surg* 2007;33(1):114–6.

36. Firoz BF, Goldberg LH, Arnon O, Mamelak AJ. An analysis of pain and analgesia after Mohs micrographic surgery. *J Am Acad Dermatol* 2010;63(1):79–86.

37. Kaplan AL, Cook JL. The incidences of chondritis and perichondritis associated with the surgical manipulation of auricular cartilage. *Dermatol Surg* 2004;30(1):58–62.

38. Maragh SL, Brown MD. Prospective evaluation of surgical site infection rate among patients with Mohs micrographic surgery without the use of prophylactic antibiotics. *J Am Acad Dermatol* 2008;59(2):275–8.

39. Mailler-Savage EA, Neal KW, Jr, Godsey T, Adams BB, Gloster HM, Jr. Is levofloxacin necessary to prevent postoperative infections of auricular second-intention wounds? *Dermatol Surg* 2008;34(1):26–30.

40. Campbell RM, Perlis CS, Fisher E, Gloster HM, Jr. Gentamicin ointment versus petrolatum for management of auricular wounds. *Dermatol Surg* 2005;31(6):664–9.

41. Rogers HD, Desciak EB, Marcus RP, Wang S, MacKay-Wiggan J, Eliezri YD. Prospective study of wound infections in Mohs micrographic surgery using clean surgical technique in the absence of prophylactic antibiotics. *J Am Acad Dermatol* 2010;63(5):842–51.

42. Dixon AJ, Dixon MP, Askew DA, Wilkinson D. Prospective study of wound infections in dermatologic surgery in the absence of prophylactic antibiotics. *Dermatol Surg* 2006;32(6):819–26.

43. Yang DJ, Quan LT, Hsu S. Topical antibacterial agents. In: Wolverton S (ed). *Comprehensive Dermatologic Drug Therapy.* 2nd ed. Philadelphia: Saunders Elsevier; 2007.

44. Onwudiwe OC, Marmur ES, Cohen JL. Are we too cavalier about antiviral prophylaxis? *J Drugs Dermatol* 2013;12(2):199–205.

45. Morales-Burgos A, Loosemore MP, Goldberg LH. Postoperative wound care after dermatologic procedures: A comparison of 2 commonly used petrolatum-based ointments. *J Drugs Dermatol* 2013;12(2):163–4.

46. Gill JF, Yu SS, Neuhaus IM. Tobacco smoking and dermatologic surgery. *J Am Acad Dermatol* 2013;68(1):167–72.

47. Ratner D. Grafts. In: Bolognia JL, Jorizzo JL, Rapini RP (eds). *Dermatology.* 2nd ed. Philadelphia: Mosby; 2008, p.2252.

48. Bowman PH, Fosko SW, Hartstein ME. Periocular reconstruction. *Semin Cutan Med Surg* 2003;22(4):263–72.

49. Goldman G, Altmayer S, Sambandan P, Cook JL. Development of cerebral air emboli during Mohs micrographic surgery. *Dermatol Surg* 2009;35(9):1414–21.

50. Sukal SA, Geronemus RG. Deep venous thrombosis following Mohs micrographic surgery: Case report. *Dermatol Surg* 2008;34(3):414–7.

PART II

Corrective Techniques in the Postoperative Period

Chapter 5

Surgical Scar Revision, Dermabrasion, and Other Physical Treatments

Ian A. Maher and Jeremy S. Bordeaux

INTRODUCTION

Scarring is a reality of all invasive cutaneous surgical procedures. This chapter will deal with the evaluation, management, and surgical and other physical revisions of facial scars that are primarily faced by Mohs and dermatological surgeons. Subsequent chapters of this book will address additional techniques available for the aesthetic improvement of surgical scars, including lasers and laser-like devices, injectable agents, and topical therapies.

Even the best-executed repairs are not completely invisible to the trained eye on close inspection. Thus, the standard that the reconstructive surgeon should aspire to is not the *absence* of scarring, but maximal *camouflage* of the scar. As discussed in the previous chapters, scar camouflage can be achieved in a number of ways. Nonetheless, all patients should be counseled prior to their surgery on the possible need for revision. The incidence of revision increases with the complexity of the repair being attempted.[1]

All surgeons will sometimes have unfortunate results that require revision. Herein we will discuss strategies for making those revisions a success. It is important to keep in mind that the first key to successful revisions is a proper initial reconstruction plan. Revisions required after well-conceptualized repairs are more often executable. On the other hand, revisions required because of repairs that were inadequately planned will be difficult, if not impossible, to successfully execute without the dreaded step of "starting over"—re-repairing the primary defect.

SCAR ANALYSIS

As the number of various scar revision procedures and tools continues to expand, their differing indications need to be considered by the surgeon. Thus, scar type analysis, as well as a thorough history and physical examination focused on scar-related findings, must be done prior to the selection of a specific revisionary technique.

History

A complete personal and family history of scarring is advisable prior to any scar revision procedure. Important findings may include a history of keloids or widened ("fish-mouth") scars; post-inflammatory hyperpigmentation; medications that inhibit wound healing, such as prednisone; and genodermatoses, such as Ehlers-Danlos syndrome, that may contribute to poor healing. Some factors, such as medication use, may be modifiable, and the surgeon should consider delaying any invasive surgical intervention until it has been stopped or the dose has been minimized. Others, such as keloid formation and post-inflammatory hyperpigmentation, are not readily modifiable, and patients should be counseled accordingly.

Physical Examination

Physical examination should focus on the specific type of the scar to be revised, as discussed below, as well as on scar location. High-tension areas, such as the chest and back, have an increased risk of keloid formaion, hypertrophy, and scar spread. The patient's other scars should also be inspected for evidence of keloids, spread, or hyperpigmentation.

Scars are complex biological entities and may simultaneously contain several of the morphologies discussed below. The order in which multiple coexistent scar characteristics are addressed has to be based on the order of their importance to the patient.

Hypertrophic and Keloidal Scars   Hypertrophic scars present as thickened fibrotic plaques limited to the area of the original wound (Figure 5.1). Hypertrophic scars may involute over time. Keloids, in contrast, are fibrotic plaques that extend beyond the boundaries of the original wound (Figure 5.2). They are frequently symptomatic—pruritic or painful—and rarely involute. They result from pathological fibroblast proliferation and collagen deposition within the wound. These scars are more common in high-tension areas, in young patients, and in darker skin types.

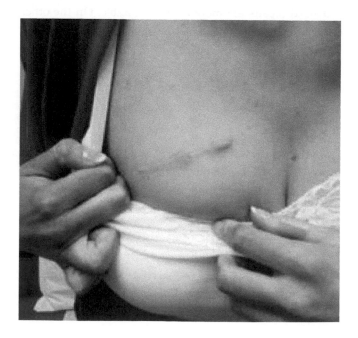

FIGURE 5.1   A hypertrophic scar on the chest following a melanoma excision.

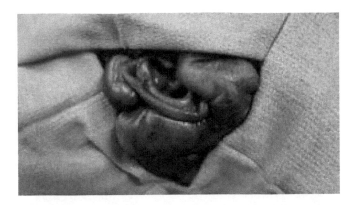

FIGURE 5.2   A large keloid on the ear.

Hypotrophic and Spread Scars   Hypotrophic scars present as depressed, and typically hypopigmented, plaques. They are wide and, in extreme cases, may approach the width of the original excision. In contrast to hypertrophic scars, these result from a paucity of collagen deposition. As mentioned in the "History" section, certain genodermatoses, may contribute to the formation of these scars. Most commonly, scar spread results from sustained wound tension or inadequate support from dermal sutures.

Inverted Scars   Inverted scars present as narrow inversions along the suture line without spread (Figure 5.3). Patients with thick, heavy, sebaceous skin have a tendency to form these scars, even when the wound edges are well everted. Such scars may also result from imprecise epidermal approximation during suturing. Inverted scars are easier to correct with minimally invasive techniques than true hypotrophic or spread scars.

Erythematous and Hyperpigmented Scars   Erythema is frequently observed in early postoperative scars (Figure 5.4).[2] This may be particularly noticeable in facial scars of patients with a tendency toward flushing or rosacea. Erythema may coexist with any other scar type. It may also lead to development of a hyperpigmented scar through the process of post-inflammatory hyperpigmentation, especially in patients with darker skin types.

Contracted Scars   Contracture is an almost universal feature of scar maturation. Placement over concave surfaces or joints can lead, respectively, to webbing or joint contracture.[3,4] Figure 5.5 shows medial canthal webbing due to contraction of a full-thickness skin graft.

Improper Tissue Volume   Inexact replacement of tissue volume may result in a less than ideal cosmetic result. This can be impossible to correct without re-repairing the primary defect. On the other hand, placement of excessive tissue in the primary defect leads to pincushioning, also called trapdoor deformity. While milder forms of pincushioning may result from other factors, such as flap edema, insufficient undermining, or ineffective deep sutures, placement of excess volume within the primary defect re-creates this problem in almost all cases.[5,6]

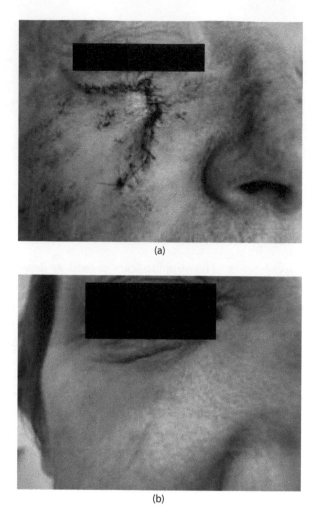

FIGURE 5.3   (a) Mohs repair of cheek defect with an advancement flap. (b) Inversion of incision lines at 6-week follow-up.

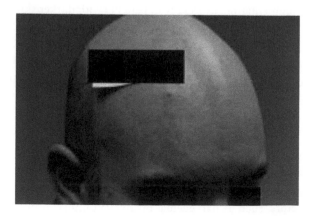

FIGURE 5.4   A patient with scar erythema after undergoing a complex linear closure on the forehead.

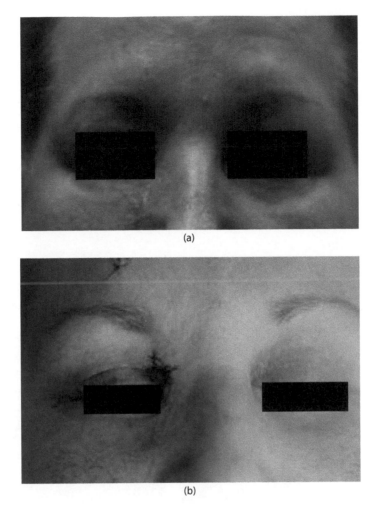

(a)

(b)

FIGURE 5.5 (a) Medial canthal webbing due to undersizing of a skin graft for medial canthal repair. (b) Repair with a Z-plasty.

SCAR REVISION TECHNIQUES
Watchful Waiting and Scar Massage

As discussed in Chapter 1, scar maturation is part of the wound healing process. Most scars undergo cosmetic improvement as they remodel over the course of 18–24 months post surgery.[7] The importance of time cannot be overestimated, and the surgeon should counsel the patient that, except in the most extreme scenarios (e.g., severe ectropion, marked oral incompetence, or a rapidly growing keloid), any surgical revision should be deferred for at least 6–8 weeks post–surgery.

Many experts advocate scar massage in the postoperative period to improve surgical scar appearance.[1] However, there is little actual high-quality data to support this maneuver.[8] It is difficult to know whether the benefits often attributed to massage may in fact be due to the natural scar maturation process. Still, massage represents a low-risk intervention. If it is undertaken, patients should be counseled to firmly rub the scar with a lubricating substance, such as petrolatum, to avoid inadvertently traumatizing the wound.

In our experience, mild versions of wound abnormalities, such as pincushioning, scar inversion, webbing, and redness, resolve over the course of 2–3 months without the need for any physician intervention. This requires patience on the part of both patient and physician. Preoperative counseling on the scar maturation process, combined with periodic review of these principles during the postoperative period, can help make the prospect of waiting more tolerable for the patient.

Once the decision to undertake a revision is made, selection of the proper revision modality is of the utmost importance.[9,10] For example, mild pincushioning is better treated with intralesional steroid injections than with surgical debulking, much as scar erythema is better targeted with pulsed dye laser treatment than with surgical or other physical resurfacing modalities. Both lasers and intralesional scar therapies will be discussed in detail in Chapters 6 and 8.

Dermabrasion

As one of the oldest scar revision technologies still employed today, dermabrasion represents a useful and cost-effective tool.[11–13] Dermabrasion relies on mechanical removal of the epidermis and superficial dermis. It can be used to flatten raised scars (Figure 5.6), blend textural

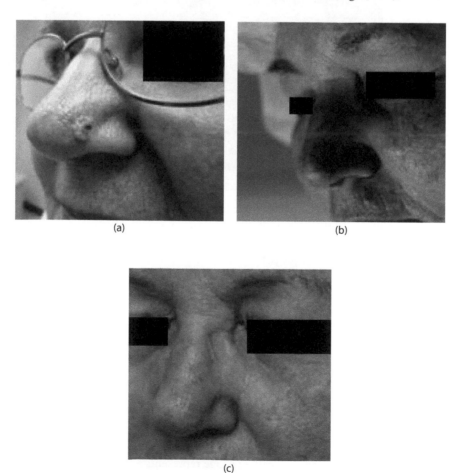

(a) (b)

(c)

FIGURE 5.6   (a) A markedly pincushioned skin graft on the nasal tip. (b) Immediately after dermabrasion. (c) Two weeks post dermabrasion, the area is completely healed, with a seamless aesthetic result.

mismatches, and attenuate depressed scar lines (Figure 5.7). While it has been suggested that dermabrasion is most useful when performed 6–8 weeks postoperatively,[14,15] dermabrasion can yield impressive improvement when delayed 3–4 months.

Dermabrasion is most effective on firm, stable skin, such as that of the nose, and should not be performed on the eyelid because of the risk of ocular injury and ectropion from scar contracture.[16] It should be approached cautiously in patients with a history of keloids and should not be performed in patients who have used oral isotretinoin in the previous 6 months,[17] though this issue has not been fully settled.[18]

Technique The area to be dermabraded should be marked with gentian violet marker. High and low areas should be marked to ascertain progress. The strategy should focus on lowering any elevated areas and on making the transitions from these into any depressed scar areas more gradual. Generally, dermabrasion should encompass at least superficial dermabrasion of the entire cosmetic subunit to improve textural uniformity. Skin

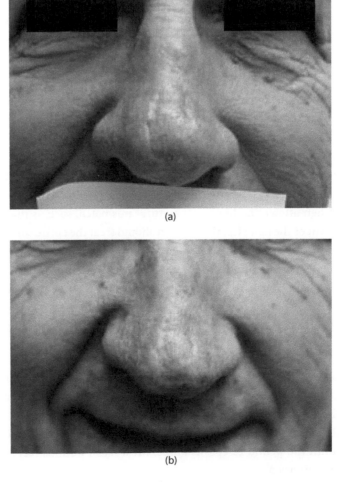

(a)

(b)

FIGURE 5.7   (a) Depressed scar lines after nasal tip repair with an island pedicle flap. (b) Improved scar blend after dermabrasion.

refrigerants have historically been used to provide anesthesia and improve the turgor of tissue to be dermabraded.[16] However, the availability of these products has waned. Instead, local anesthesia with injectable lidocaine with epinephrine provides effective anesthesia for the localized dermabrasion while increasing skin turgor.

Once the area is marked and anesthetized, it should be prepped with an appropriate surgical disinfectant, such as betadine or chlorhexidine. Both patient and staff should don impervious gowns and eye and hair protection to prevent communication of blood-borne disease and soilage of clothing by the tissue debris created by mechanical dermabrasion. Dermabrasion may be performed with a mechanical hand engine, such as those manufactured by Bell Handengine®, Inc. (Grants Pass, OR) or Osada, Inc. (Los Angeles, CA),[16,17] though equivalent efficacy has been demonstrated with manual dermabrasion with sterilized sandpaper.[19,20] Our preference is to use the Bell hand engine with a diamond fraise, as it allows for rapid, consistent, and predictable resurfacing.

The hand engine should be held in the dominant hand with a pencil grip. Most mechanical dermabraders feature a foot switch. The fraise should encounter the skin at a 30°–45° angle. The long axis of the handle should be kept perpendicular to any free margins. If the handle is oriented parallel to a free margin and the direction of rotation of the fraise is away from the free margin, the tissue can be inadvertently drawn together by the dermabrader, leading to injury to unintended areas (e.g., tooth enamel when dermabrading the upper lip).

With the fraise and handle in proper orientation just above the area to be dermabraded, the foot switch can be actuated and the spinning tip brought into contact with the tissue. The fraise should be kept constantly moving over the area with a gentle back-and-forth or circular motion to prevent burrowing or gouging of the tip into the tissue. Elevated areas should be gradually sanded down to the level of the normal tissue. When treating depressed scars, the surgeon should sand the areas *around* the depressed scar to attenuate the transition to the normal tissue. When attempting to correct textural mismatch, such as that between a skin graft and native skin of the nasal tip, the surgeon should treat the entire subunit until confluent punctate bleeding is seen. When needed, an assistant may utilize saline–moistened gauze to wipe away any debris from the field to improve visualization. It is of prime importance that gauze, drapes, hair, clothes, and other loose materials be kept well away from the rotating dermabrader tip, as entanglement could result in injury to the patient, staff, or surgeon, as well as almost certain damage to the instrument.

Postoperative Care   Significant oozing may occur during and after dermabrasion. Applying gauze pad moistened with 3 mL of lidocaine with epinephrine for 2–3 minutes is generally effective in producing vasoconstriction and hemostasis. Ointment and a pressure dressing can then be applied. This dressing is left intact for 24–48 hours. The patient is then instructed to perform daily wound cleaning with gentle soap, followed by application of ointment and a bandage until the wound re-epithelializes. Most facial wounds reepithelialize within 5–7 days post dermabrasion.

Surgical Scar Revision

There are numerous surgical scar revision techniques with wide ranges of indications. Selection of the appropriate procedure to correct the problem at hand is of the utmost importance when this type of revision is considered. Except in cases of true function-limiting scars (e.g., severe ectropion, oral incompetence), surgical scar revision is best delayed 6–12 months after the original surgery to allow for scar maturation.

Direct Scar Excision   Direct scar excision is the simplest surgical revisionary procedure (Figure 5.8). An inverted, spread, or keloidal scar may be excised in an elliptical manner and closed linearly.[21] Though keloid excision is a complicated topic unto itself and will not

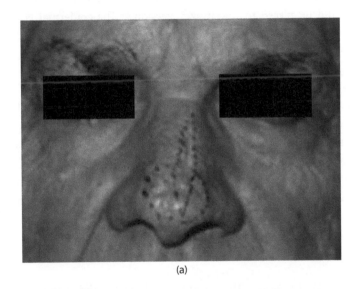

(a)

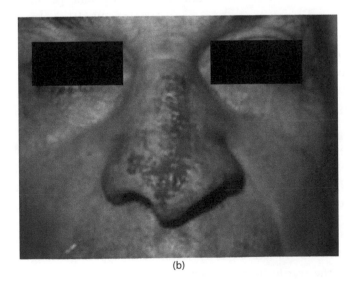

(b)

FIGURE 5.8   (a) Planned scar excision. (b) After scar excision.

be discussed in detail here, adjunct use of intralesional steroids, as discussed in Chapter 8, may be considered in such cases. Before the procedure, careful analysis of the root cause of the undesirable result must be performed. As previously discussed, scars on high-tension areas, such as the upper trunk and proximal extremities, have a natural tendency to spread. Alternatively, a patient may have a history of spread or atrophic scars, which makes it likely that the same result will be seen after a revisionary procedure.

If scar excision is to be performed, an ellipse is marked around the scar. Once anesthesia is achieved, the scar is excised. Some authors advocate leaving a small amount of scar tissue in the wound bed to add bulk and to prevent re-inversion of the scar.[22] Wide undermining should be performed to minimize tension on the wound edges. Buried vertical mattress sutures should be placed to maximize eversion.[23] The epidermal edges should then be carefully re-approximated. This type of revision relies entirely on meticulous surgical technique to deliver an outcome superior to that of the original procedure. Such being the case, great care should be taken intraoperatively.

Debulking   Debulking, such as for a pincushioned transposition flap, can be thought of as a three-dimensional version of scar excision. Instead of marking an ellipse around the scar, the surgeon marks the original incision lines along with the areas of excess tissue volume. After anesthesia is achieved, the original incision lines are re-incised in the area of the pincushioning defect to access the extra bulk. Excess subdermal fibrofatty tissue is excised to correct the contour discrepancy. Meticulous hemostasis prevents hematoma formation in this new potential space, which could otherwise lead to recurrence of the contour deformity. The area is widely undermined, and high-quality buried vertical mattress sutures are placed to prevent recurrence of the trapdoor defect.

Scar Disruption Techniques   The running W-plasty and geometric broken line closure may be used as adjuncts to scar excision. In a W-plasty, the opposing wound edges are trimmed in an opposing zigzag manner, so that when brought together, they fit together in a tongue-and-groove pattern. The running geometric broken line closure involves cutting the opposing wound edges in random geometric shapes (Figure 5.9). It is also designed so that the edges, when apposed, fit in a tongue-in-groove pattern. Both closures seek to break a visible scar into shorter segments, which are less perceptible.[24] These scar disruption techniques are useful for the same groups of scars as direct scar excision, and they have the added value of being able to reorient portions of a malpositioned scar into the relaxed skin tension lines (RSTLs) (see Figure 2.2).[25] The same meticulous patient selection and surgical technique are required for these modifications as for direct scar excision.

Scar Reorientation   Z-plasty is the classic example of a surgical revision to reorient scars and redistribute tension. Z-plasty creates two opposing triangular flaps, whose common side is the scar to be reoriented (Figure 5.10). When the flaps are transposed over one another, the central scar is reoriented.[24] Due to the length exchange between the shorter central limb and the larger distance between the bases of the triangular flaps,

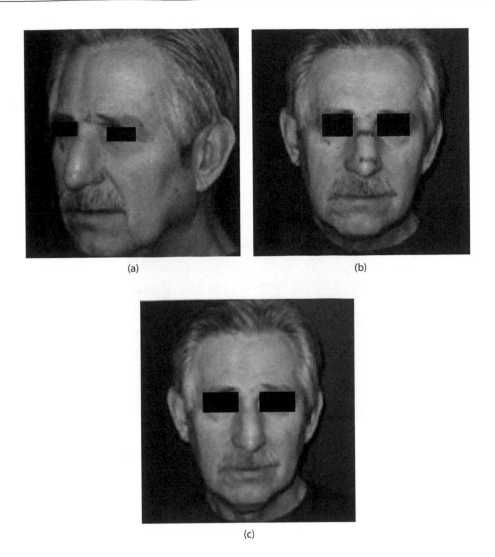

(a)   (b)

(c)

FIGURE 5.9   (a) Visible suture lines at the distal and proximal margins of inset of a paramedian forehead flap. (b) Planned geometric broken line closure. (c) Final result.

the scar is lengthened (Figure 5.11). Thus, the Z-plasty may be used not only to reorient a malpositioned scar but also to obtain tension release in a contracted scar. Z-plasty may be used to reposition a retracted free margin, correct webbing of a scar over a concavity, or release a contracted joint.

Z-plasty design can be confusing even for an experienced surgeon. Remembering several key points makes it more accessible (Table 5.1). Once designed, the area is anesthetized and prepped. The incisions are made, and the area is widely undermined to release scar contracture and to allow for tension-free closure. The flaps are then transposed into the new orientation and carefully sutured to maximize camouflage of the newly created suture lines. Placing

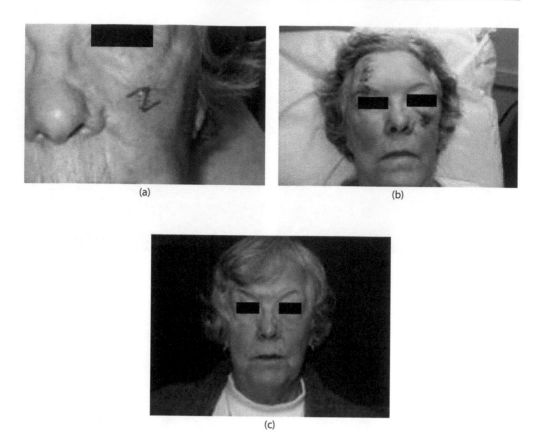

FIGURE 5.10   (a) Z-plasty to reorient a scar on the cheek. (b) Sutured result. (c) Final result.

a dot on one of the triangular flaps can help ensure that the flaps are sutured into their correct final orientation.[21]

A V-Y flap is an advancement flap that can be used to "push" a distorted free margin into place or to release a contracted scar.[24,26] A V-shaped incision is made through the dermis. Undermining is performed around the scar but, most importantly, not beneath the newly created triangular flap of tissue. The trailing edge of the "V" is closed linearly, pushing the flap into its desired position. The mathematical principles underlying the V-Y flap have not been explored as rigorously as those of the Z-plasty. The lengthening effect of the V-Y advancement results from the pushing vector generated by closure of the secondary defect at the trailing edge of the flap. It is generally not as effective in producing lengthening as the Z-plasty and is therefore used less frequently.

Not to be confused with the V-Y closure, a Y-V flap may be used to pull a free margin that has been distorted by a pushing vector (e.g., a downwardly distorted upper vermilion border or a "bulldozed" alar margin). A Y-shaped incision is made above the free margin to be reoriented, with the long axis of the "Y" placed perpendicularly to the free margin. The V-shaped

60 degree Z-Plasty before transposition

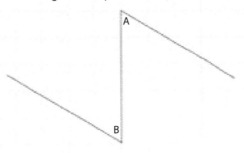

60 degree Z-plasty after transposition

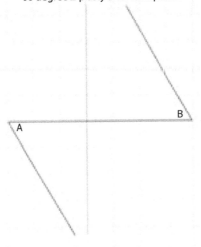

FIGURE 5.11 A schematic of a 60° Z-plasty. The scar to be elongated is marked with a solid red line. The elongated final length is signified by the red dotted line. A 60° Z-plasty produces 75% scar lengthening.

TABLE 5.1   Z-Plasty Technique

1. The central limb is the scar to be released/reoriented.
2. From either end of the central limb, mirror-image peripheral limbs are drawn in opposite directions from the opposite ends of the scar. For a single Z-plasty, the lengths of the peripheral limbs should equal the length of the central limb.
3. The angle at which these peripheral limbs intersect with the central limb determines the degree of lengthening. The greater the angle of incidence, the more the lengthening (Figure 5.11).
4. For each central limb, two different mirror-image Z-plasties can be designed. The resulting scar orientation can be anticipated by visualizing a line that connects the bases of the two flaps. The Z-plasty that places the final scars into the most advantageous orientation should be selected.
5. In the case of a longer scar, where a single large Z-plasty would be impossible, the scar may be broken up into segments and addressed by a series of smaller Z-plasties. These follow the same design principles as a single Z-plasty.

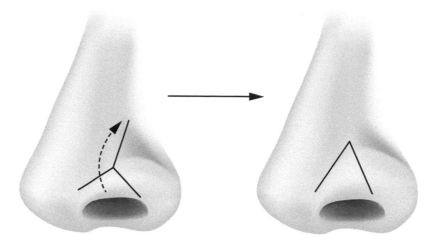

FIGURE 5.12   A Y-V flap may be used to elevate a free margin.

scar is created by advancing the apex toward the base of the Y until the desired margin retraction is achieved (Figure 5.12).[27]

CHEMICAL SCAR RESURFACING AND OTHER PHYSICAL MODALITIES

Other physical treatments utilizing various chemical peels and microneedling devices, such as Dermaroller (Dermaroller GmbH, Wolfenbüttel, Germany) or DermaStamp (Lamelle, Sandton, South Africa), have been successfully used in the treatment of various atrophic scars, such as acne and varicella scars.[28-31] These techniques rely on injury-provoked neocollagenesis and the production of ground substance to normalize the appearance of scars.[32] Unfortunately, studies evaluating these modalities in the treatment of postsurgical or post-Mohs scars are lacking; this would be an important future research topic.

Additionally, a technique known as chemical reconstruction of skin scars (CROSS) has been described in literature.[33-35] The procedure involves pinpoint application of concentrated acid, such as 80%–100% trichrolacetic acid, to the base of an atrophic scar using a sharpened wooden applicator. This results in the immediate frosting of the base, followed in several days by desiccation and eventually by sloughing off of the epidermal tissue. This is thought to stimulate new collagenogenesis, which gradually results in the elevation of the scar base.[35] Several sessions, typically performed 2–4 weeks apart, may be required for optimal improvement. While this technique also has not been formally studied in the context of post-Mohs surgical scars, anecdotal evidence suggests its potential usefulness in the treatment of small depressed scars, such as those occasionally encountered following second intent healing (Figure 5.13).

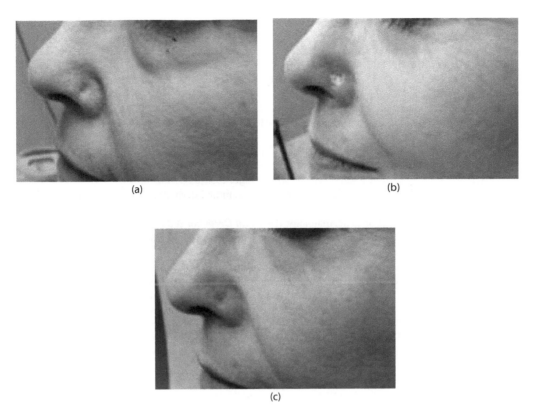

FIGURE 5.13 A depressed scar treated with the CROSS technique using 95% TCA. The patient underwent Mohs surgery for a basal cell carcinoma but did not want a repair after tumor extirpation. (a) Atrophic scar before TCA-CROSS. (b) Immediate frosting upon application. (c) Appearance after two sessions. Note that the scar is shallower. (Courtesy of Alexander L. Berlin, M.D.)

CONCLUSIONS

Scar revision is an inevitable part of the Mohs or dermatological surgeon's practice. The ability to properly analyze scars allows the surgeon to select the proper scar revision modality. Optimum results can be achieved by pairing a specific scar type with the appropriate scar revision modality.

REFERENCES

1. Menick FJ. Nasal reconstruction. *Plast Reconstr Surg* 2010;125(4):138e–50e.
2. Elsaie ML, Choudhary S. Lasers for scars: A review and evidence-based appraisal. *J Drugs Dermatol* 2010;9:1355–62.
3. Massry GG. Cicatricial canthal webs. *Ophthal Plast Reconstr Surg* 2011;27(6):426–30.
4. Grishkevich VM. Flexion contractures of fingers: Contracture elimination with trapeze-flap plasty. *Burns* 2011;37(1):126–33.
5. Zitelli JA. Modification of the Zitelli bilobed flap: A comparison of flap dynamics in human cadavers (comment). *Arch Facial Plast Surg* 2006;8(6):410.
6. Xue C, Li L, Guo L, Li J, Xing X. The bilobed flap for reconstruction of distal nasal defect in Asians. *Aesthetic Plast Surg* 2009;33(4):600–4.
7. Clark RA. Biology of dermal wound repair. *Dermatol Clin* 1993;11(4):647–66.

8. Shin TM, Bordeaux JS. The role of massage in scar management: A literature review. *Dermatol Surg* 2012;38(3):414–23.
9. Koranda FC, Webster RC. Trapdoor effect in nasolabial flaps. Causes and corrections. *Arch Otolaryngol* 1985;111(7):421–4.
10. Chang CW, Ries WR. Nonoperative techniques for scar management and revision. *Facial Plast Surg* 2001;17(4):283–8.
11. Roenigk HH. Dermabrasion: State of the art 2002. *J Cosmet Dermatol* 2002;1(2):7287.
12. Lawrence N, Mandy S, Yarborough J, Alt T. History of dermabrasion. *Dermatol Surg* 2000;26(2):95–101.
13. Hruza GJ. Dermabrasion. *Facial Plast Surg Clin North Am* 2001;9(2):267–81, ix.
14. Katz BE, Oca AG. A controlled study of the effectiveness of spot dermabrasion ("scarabrasion") on the appearance of surgical scars. *J Am Acad Dermatol* 1991;24(3):462–6.
15. Yarborough JM Jr. Ablation of facial scars by programmed dermabrasion. *J Dermatol Surg Oncol* 1988;14(3):292–4.
16. Gold MH. Dermabrasion in dermatology. *Am J Clin Dermatol* 2003;4(7):467–71.
17. Surowitz JB, Shockley WW. Enhancement of facial scars with dermabrasion. *Facial Plast Surg Clin North Am* 2011(3);19:517–25.
18. Bagatin E, dos Santos Guadanhim LR, Yarak S, Kamamoto CS, de Almeida FA. Dermabrasion for acne scars during treatment with oral isotretinoin. *Dermatol Surg* 2010;36(4):483–9.
19. Poulos E, Taylor C, Solish N. Effectiveness of dermasanding (manual dermabrasion) on the appearance of surgical scars: A prospective, randomized, blinded study. *J Am Acad Dermatol* 2003;48(6):897–900.
20. Gillard M, Wang TS, Boyd CM, Dunn RL, Fader DJ, Johnson TM. Conventional diamond fraise vs manual spot dermabrasion with drywall sanding screen for scars from skin cancer surgery. *Arch Dermatol* 2002;138(8):1035–9.
21. Lee KK, Mehrany K, Swanson NA. Surgical revision. *Dermatol Clin* 2005;23(1):141–50, vii.
22. Harahap M. Revision of a depressed scar. *J Dermatol Surg Oncol* 1984;10(3):206–9.
23. Zitelli JA, Moy RL. Buried vertical mattress suture. *J Dermatol Surg Oncol* 1989;15(1):17–9.
24. Shockley WW. Scar revision techniques: Z-plasty, W-plasty, and geometric broken line closure. *Facial Plast Surg Clin North Am* 2011;19(3):455–63.
25. Borges AF. Relaxed skin tension lines (RSTL) versus other skin lines. *Plast Reconstr Surg* 1984;73(1):144–50.
26. Askar I. Double reverse V-Y-plasty in postburn scar contractures: A new modification of V-Y-plasty. *Burns* 2003;29(7):721–5.
27. van Niekerk WJ, Taggart I. The size of the Y: The multiple Y-V plasty revisited. *Burns* 2008;34(2):257–61.
28. Monheit GD. The Jessner's-trichloroacetic acid peel. An enhanced medium-depth chemical peel. *Dermatol Clin* 1995;13(2):277–83.
29. Garg VK, Sinha S, Sarkar R. Glycolic acid peels versus salicylic-mandelic acid peels in active acne vulgaris and post-acne scarring and hyperpigmentation: A comparative study. *Dermatol Surg* 2009;35(1):59–65.
30. Leheta T, El Tawdy A, Abdel Hay R, Farid S. Percutaneous collagen induction versus full-concentration trichloroacetic acid in the treatment of atrophic acne scars. *Dermatol Surg* 2011;37(2):207–16.
31. Sharad J. Combination of microneedling and glycolic acid peels for the treatment of acne scars in dark skin. *J Cosmet Dermatol* 2011;10(4):317–23.
32. Kim SE, Lee JH, Kwon HB, Ahn BJ, Lee AY. Greater collagen deposition with the microneedle therapy system than with intense pulsed light. *Dermatol Surg* 2011;37(3):336–41.
33. Lee JB, Chung WG, Kwahck H, Lee KH. Focal treatment of acne scars with trichloroacetic acid: Chemical reconstruction of skin scars method. *Dermatol Surg* 2002;28(11):1017–21.
34. Cho SB, Park CO, Chung WG, Lee KH, Lee JB, Chung KY. Histometric and histochemical analysis of the effect of trichloroacetic acid concentration in the chemical reconstruction of skin scars method. *Dermatol Surg* 2006;32(10):1231–6.
35. Yug A, Lane JE, Howard MS, Kent DE. Histologic study of depressed acne scars treated with serial high-concentration (95%) trichloroacetic acid. *Dermatol Surg* 2006;32(8):985–90.

Chapter 6

Lasers and Laser-Like Devices

Lara K. Butler, Irene J. Vergilis, and Joel L. Cohen

INTRODUCTION

In addition to the physical therapies discussed in the previous chapter, laser scar revision has now gained recognition for its safety profile and clinically demonstrable efficacy. A multitude of laser and laser-like devices are currently available for the improvement of scars. These devices are broken down into the following technologies: ablative, nonablative, and fractional. The three types differ in their method of action and in the extent of thermal damage, length of downtime, adverse effect profile, and efficacy.

Laser therapy may improve the appearance of wounded skin by promoting better collagen organization in healing wounds.[1] In addition, it has been suggested that combination therapy using lasers and other treatment modalities discussed in other chapters further improves long-term scar revision.[2] However, no consensus is available in the literature as to what constitutes optimal therapy.

OPTIMAL TIME TO TREAT

Acute optimization of wound healing can start immediately after the completion of surgery, as in laser-assisted scar healing (LASH);[3] following suture removal; or several weeks to months after surgery, when the scar has matured. As early as 1956, Strauss and Kligman reported that dermabrasion of the wound edges at the time of closure improved the final cosmesis of sutured wounds.[4] Similarly, in the past two decades, several studies using ablative and nonablative laser devices on surgical wounds at the time of closure have shown promising trends in improvement of scar appearance and texture.[5–8] In theory, earlier intervention can alter the inflammatory phase of wound healing and affect fibroblast migration, thus leading to reduced scarring.

NONABLATIVE LASER AND LIGHT THERAPIES
Pulsed Dye Laser

Developed in the early 1990s, the flashlamp-pumped 585 nm and 595 nm pulsed dye lasers (PDLs) became the standard of care in the treatment of vascular lesions such as capillary malformations (i.e., port wine stains) and facial telangiectases. This vascular-specific laser works via selective photothermolysis that targets blood vessels, thereby minimizing collateral damage. The energy from the PDL is preferentially absorbed by hemoglobin, resulting in local thermal injury in the papillary and reticular dermis at the level of the microvasculature. Thrombosis, vasculitis, and gradual repair follow. Although there is no consensus regarding the mechanism by which PDL affects scarring, it has been postulated that destruction of microvascular blood supply leads to ischemia, which may affect collagen synthesis or collagenase release or deprive a scar of nutrients, thereby preventing scar hypertrophy.[9] Therefore, early intervention with PDL may control the degree of angiogenesis and extinguish the hypervascular response.[10]

Over the past two decades, the efficacy of PDL therapy for the treatment of hypertrophic and keloid scars has been studied extensively. These devices have been shown to reduce scar volume, pruritus, and pain and to improve texture, color, and pliability. Both 585 nm and 595 nm wavelengths have been demonstrated to improve cosmesis; however, 585 nm has been suggested to be the preferred wavelength, since it substantially normalizes scar height in addition to vascularity and pliability.[11] Although several studies have actually shown PDL to be ineffective in scar reduction, numerous factors may have led to contradictory results, including location, skin type, outcome measurement methods, laser settings, and follow-up duration.[12,13]

Proposed PDL parameters (Table 6.1) for treatment of hypertrophic scars and keloids in skin types I–III include pulse durations ranging from 0.45 to 1.5 ms and fluences of 4.5–5.5 J /cm^2 (10 mm spot), 6.0–7.0 J/cm^2 (7 mm spot), or 6.5–7.5 J/cm^2 (5 mm spot), with overlapping pulses. Reevaluation is typically performed in 6–8 weeks.[10,14] Parameters may vary based on the size and thickness of the scar. Because melanin competes with hemoglobin as a chromophore, use of the PDL may not be as effective in patients with skin types IV, V, and VI.[15] To avoid complications, energy densities should be lowered by at least 0.5 J/cm^2 for darker-skinned patients and for scars in thin-skinned areas (eyelids, chest, and neck).

Studies have shown that most hypertrophic scars require an average of two treatments with either PDL device to achieve 50%–80% improvement (Figure 6.1).[16–18] Keloid scars are more fibrotic and consequently require additional treatments to achieve similar results. A wealth of published clinical data over the past two decades has revealed that PDL is the laser of choice for treating hypertrophic and keloid scars[14] or, quite simply, scars with excessive erythema or neovascularization.

TABLE 6.1   Recommendations for Laser- and Light-Based Scar Revision

Scar Type	Laser	Settings	Adverse Effects
Hypertrophic & keloid	PDL (585 or 595 nm)	6.0–7.5 J/cm^2 (7 mm spot) or 4.5–5.5 J/cm^2 (10 mm spot), 0.45–1.5 ms, overlapping pulses (parameters vary based on the size and thickness of the scar)	Transient purpura (several days to 1 week), edema, hyperpigmentation
	CO$_2$ (10 600 nm)	1 pass, 250–350 mJ, 60 W, 5 J/cm^2	Erythema, edema, and drainage (weeks-months)
	Er:YAG (2940 nm)	2–3 passes, 5 mm spot, 5–15 J/cm^2	Erythema, edema, and drainage (weeks)
	Nonablative fractional (1540/1550 nm)	15 mm handpiece, 35–50 J/cm^2	Transient erythema and edema
Atrophic	CO$_2$ (10 600 nm)	1 pass, 250–350 mJ, 60 W, 5 J/cm^2	Erythema, edema and drainage (weeks–months)
	Er:YAG (2940 nm)	2–3 passes, 5 mm spot, 5 –15 J/cm^2	Erythema, edema and drainage (weeks)
	Er:glass (1540 nm)	4 mm spot, 8–10 J/cm^2, 3 ms	Minimal erythema and edema (hours)
	Diode (1450 nm)	6 mm spot, 8–14 J/cm^2, 250 ms	Minimal erythema and edema (hours)
	Nd:YAG (1320 nm)	6 mm spot, 18 J/cm^2, 200 ms	Minimal erythema and edema (hours)

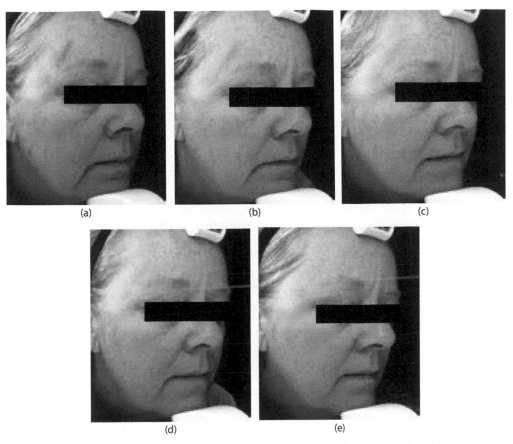

FIGURE 6.1 Surgical scar: (a) Before treatment, at 4-5 weeks after surgery. (b–d) During treatment with 595 nm PDL (VBeam Perfecta, Candela, Wayland, MA) using 10 mm spot size, fluence of 7.5 J/ cm², pulse duration of 3 ms, and one pass. (e) After four treatments at 6 week intervals. Notice significant improvement in color and texture of the scar visible after just two sessions. (Courtesy of Joel L. Cohen, Colorado, USA.)

PDL is generally well tolerated, with few adverse effects reported other than posttreatment purpura. Pulse durations of less than 6 ms are almost certain to cause bruising of the skin, which typically lasts 7–10 days. Edema of the treated area may also occur but usually subsides within 48 hours. Strict sun avoidance and diligent photo-protection should be advocated between treatment sessions to avoid hyperpigmentation, which has been reported in the literature with varying frequencies (1%–24%).[19] Although good clinical results have been observed with PDL irradiation of scars, post-treatment purpura persisting for several days somewhat limits its usefulness for nonablative resurfacing.

Concomitant use of intralesional corticosteroids or 5-fluorouracil with PDL has been shown to provide additional benefit in proliferative scars.[2,20] Intralesional injections of corticosteroids (20 mg/mL or 40 mg/mL of triamcinolone acetonide [Kenalog', Bristol-Myers Squibb, New York, NY]) are more easily delivered after PDL irradiation because the ensuing edema, allowing easier needle penetration.[20] The use of concomitant high-energy pulsed CO_2 and PDL laser systems was found to be superior to use of CO_2 laser vaporization alone for revision of non-erythematous hypertrophic scars (Figures 6.2 and 6.3).[21] Research continues to

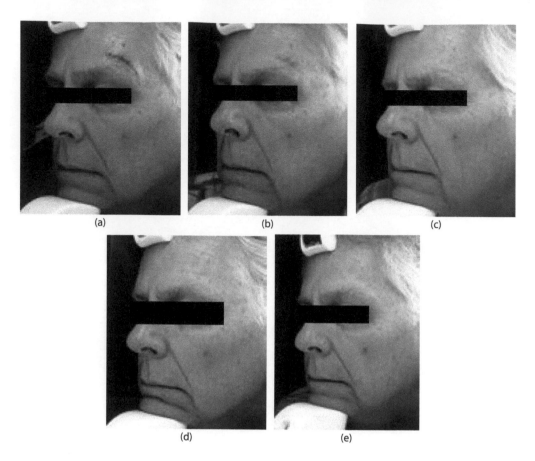

FIGURE 6.2 Combination therapy with 595 nm PDL (VBeam Perfecta, Candela, Wayland, MA) and ablative fractionated CO_2 laser (CO_2RE, Syneron-Candela, Irvine, CA) starting on the day of suture removal. PDL was used with a 10 mm spot size, fluence of 7.5 J/cm², pulse duration of 3 ms, and one pass. Ablative fractionated CO_2 laser was used at the following settings: First treatment: 25% fractional coverage, Ring104 CORE 70; second through fourth treatments: 30% fractional coverage, Ring 104 CORE 70. (a) Postoperative scar from skin cancer surgery. (b–d) During treatment with combination PDL and AFL. (e) After 4 treatment sessions, with significant improvement in appearance of surgical scar. (Courtesy of Joel L. Cohen, Colorado, USA.)

suggest that the vascular specificity of the PDL, whether used alone or in combination with other modalities, is linked to improvement in hypertrophic scar tissue. [2,20,21]

Other Nonablative Lasers

Newer-generation nonablative lasers (long-pulsed 1320 nm Nd:YAG, 1450 nm diode, and 1540 nm erbium:glass) have yielded inconsistent results for revision of scars.[10,22] These devices deliver deeply penetrating infrared wavelengths, which target tissue water and stimulate collagen production via controlled dermal heating coupled with protective epidermal cooling. These systems have been mostly studied mostly in the treatment of atrophic acne scars, with mild to moderate clinical improvement (40%–50%) appreciated several months after undergoing a series of three to five monthly treatments at monthly intervals.[22–24] Relative to conventional ablative lasers, the low side effect profile and more rapid recovery may compensate for their lesser clinical efficacy.

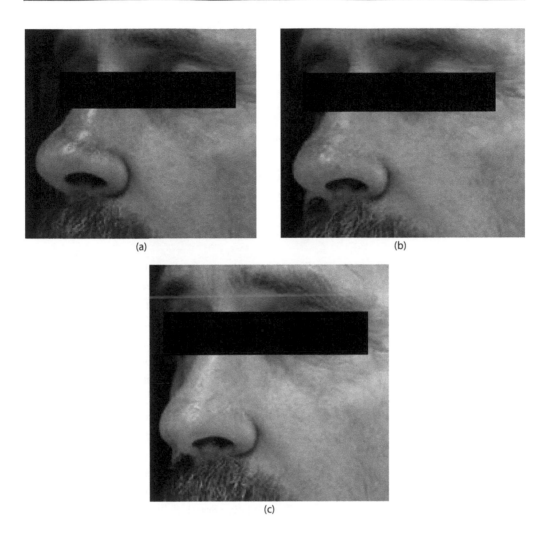

(a)   (b)

(c)

FIGURE 6.3   Combination therapy with ablative fractionated 2940 nm Er:YAG laser (ProFractional, Sciton, Palo Alto, CA) and 595 nm PDL (VBeam Perfecta, Candela, Wayland, MA). (a) Scar at 8 weeks after skin cancer surgery. (b) After one treatment using fractional Er:YAG at 200 J/cm^2, Coag2, 22% fractional coverage, and two passes. (c) After two more treatments with Er:YAG plus two treatments with PDL using 10 mm spot size, 6 ms pulse duration, and 8 J/cm^2 of fluence. (Courtesy of Joel L. Cohen, Colorado, USA.)

Intense Pulsed Light

Intense pulsed light (IPL) devices deliver focused, controlled light energy across the 515–1200 nm spectrum through a coupling gel. Specific filters in the handpiece block lower wavelengths and allow the user to select a specific therapeutic window, such as 755 nm to stimulate collagen synthesis, 695 nm to minimize superficial leg veins, or 515 nm to treat erythema of rosacea. However, the exact mechanism of action is unknown.

Traditionally, IPL has been used for cosmetic purposes. It has also been shown to help in management of the dyschromia and hypervascularity associated with many scars without the risks or downtime of the PDL photothermolysis or ablative laser resurfacing devices discussed below. Several reports in the literature have demonstrated significant improvement in hypertrophic and keloid scar thickness, erythema, and firmness after treatment with IPL.[25,26] Thus, IPL may offer another method of treating scars that minimizes the risk of purpura.

No significant negative long-term effects have been observed with IPL. However, caution must be exercised on hair-bearing skin, such as beard or mustache areas in male patients, as well as arms and legs, since hair removal may result from treatment. Additionally, in order to avert unnecessary worry or concerns, patients should be warned that pigmented lesions, such as lentigos and ephelides, may temporarily darken prior to their sloughing and eventual lightening.

Excimer Laser for Hypopigmentation

Hypopigmented scars can occur as a direct consequence of cutaneous surgery or as a side effect of ablative and fractional resurfacing, as discussed in the sections "Ablative Laser Therapy" and "Ablative Fractional Lasers." Prior to the introduction of the single-wavelength 308 nm excimer laser, treatments for such scars had limited efficacy and variable safety profiles. Based on the finding that narrowband ultraviolet B (UVB) light (311–312 nm) has been effective in repigmenting vitiligo,[27–29] it was theorized that the 308 nm excimer laser might also correct hypopigmentation by increasing melanin production. A prior case study showed that this laser may be used to treat post-resurfacing leukoderma.[30] More recently, it was shown to be a safe and effective method for pigment correction of hypopigmented scars.[31] However, a major limitation to this therapeutic intervention is the need for multiple sessions initially, as well as maintenance treatments every 1–4 months to maintain cosmetic benefit. Optimal treatment parameters need to be established in future studies. An additional, novel combination treatment involving a laser and a topical agent for the improvement of hypopigmentation will be discussed in the section "Nonablative Fractional Lasers."

ABLATIVE LASER THERAPY

Ablative laser resurfacing offers a highly efficacious treatment modality for scar revision, as it allows for the complete removal of the epidermis and parts of the dermis. In addition, it stimulates wound remodeling with new collagen formation and subsequent improvement in atrophic scars. Since the concept of fractional photothermolysis was introduced almost a decade ago, the use of these conventional fully ablative lasers has become less common. Interestingly, the pendulum may be starting to swing back, as many physicians are finding fully ablative lasers to be much more effective for resurfacing rhytids in the perioral and periocular areas. As a consequence, these lasers are increasingly pursued for scar revision despite a greater side effect profile.

Ablative CO_2 and erbium:YAG (Er:YAG) lasers selectively heat and vaporize superficial skin by emitting energy that is absorbed by intracellular water. The depth of ablation correlates directly with the fluence as well as with the number of passes and is usually confined to the epidermis and papillary dermis. It should be noted, however, that stacking laser pulses by performing multiple passes in rapid succession or by using a high overlap setting on a scanning device can penetrate much deeper into the skin, increasing the risk of scarring. Although spot vaporization of isolated scars is a practical therapeutic option, extending treatment to involve the entire cosmetic subunit has been recommended to help avoid unwanted lines of demarcation.[14] Lighter settings can then be used to feather out or blend treatment zones more gradually.

Despite their clinical efficacy, fully ablative resurfacing lasers have lost some momentum due to problems with precision, prolonged recovery times, erythema, and posttreatment pigmentary alterations.[32,33] The short-pulsed Er:YAG laser was designed as the less ablative alternative to the CO_2 laser.[34] This device emits a 2940 nm wavelength, which is closer to the peak absorption of water. At this wavelength, light is absorbed 12–18 times more efficiently by superficial aqueous tissue than it is at the 10,600 nm wavelength of the CO_2 laser.[35] Consequently, tissue ablation is more precise and residual thermal damage is reduced, resulting in shorter recovery times and a more favorable side effect profile.[36,37] On the other hand, compared to the CO_2 laser device, the short-pulsed Er:YAG laser produces more modest intraoperative hemostasis, less collagen contraction, and less striking clinical improvement.[37,38] The dual-mode Er:YAG laser was designed to overcome these limitations. This device produces both ablative and coagulative pulses and produces greater collagen contraction, deeper tissue vaporization, and improved hemostasis.[39]

The ideal patient for ablative laser skin resurfacing has an atrophic scar and a fair complexion (skin phototype I or II). Absolute contraindications include active bacterial, viral, or fungal infection, active inflammatory skin condition (e.g., psoriasis, eczema) in the treatment area, isotretinoin use in the past 6 months, and history of keloids. The recommended settings for ablative CO_2 and Er:YAG lasers can be found in Table 6.1. Compared to the CO_2 laser, the short-pulsed Er:YAG often requires several passes to achieve a similar depth of penetration, whereas the long-pulsed Er:YAG laser is operated at higher fluences to achieve comparable results in a single pass.[14]

Most atrophic scars require at least two passes regardless of the laser system. It is important to remove any partially desiccated tissue with saline- or water-soaked gauze between passes, to prevent char formation. Areas of thinner skin (e.g., periorbital) require fewer laser passes.

Postoperative wound care is critical, and patients should be provided with both verbal and written instructions. It should be noted that while plain topical ointments and semi-occlusive dressings promote healing, topical antibiotics may cause contact dermatitis and should be avoided.[40] Following ablative laser resurfacing, the vaporized skin usually takes 7–10 days to reepithelialize. Treated areas appear erythematous and edematous, with serosanguinous discharge. Postoperative erythema typically lasts 4–6 weeks following treatment with the Er:YAG laser but may persist for up to 3–4 months with the CO_2 laser. Transient hyperpigmentation commonly appears 3–4 weeks after treatment, while delayed-onset permanent hypopigmentation can be seen months later in about one-fifth of patients.[33]

Overly aggressive laser techniques can cause hypertrophic scarring and lead to ectropion formation in the periorbital area. In addition, fully ablative laser resurfacing of the face should either be performed with low settings and extreme caution or avoided altogether. This is due to the high risk for scarring at these locations, which is related to the relative paucity of pilosebaceous units. Treatment of large areas and of periorificial skin often necessitates the use of prophylactic antibiotics or antiviral medications to reduce the risk for infection and subsequent scarring.[41,42]

To optimize scar revision success, it is imperative that patients be closely monitored for potential complications, such as infections and contact dermatitis, for the first month after the treatment.

FRACTIONAL LASER THERAPY

The newest laser technology to enter the field of resurfacing is fractional photothermolysis (FP). Since its introduction in 2007, fractional laser resurfacing has been largely used for cosmetic indications, such as treatment of photoaging, fine rhytids of the mouth and eyelids, and abnormal pigmentation. Over the past decade, fractional laser resurfacing has also emerged as a popular and effective means of treating surgical scars.

Fractional laser systems can be classified into two categories: ablative fractional lasers (AFLs) and nonablative fractional lasers (NAFLs).[14] These devices emit pixelated light, producing microthermal zones (MTZs) that are typically 70–100 μm in diameter and 250–800 μm in depth. This results in small columns of thermally altered skin with intervening islands of normal tissue, which rapidly repopulate the ablated areas.[43] MTZs in AFLs extend through the epidermis and dermis, while NAFLs leave the stratum corneum intact. Maintainance of the stratum corneum ensures continuous epidermal barrier function while allowing for localized subcorneal epidermal necrosis and dermal matrix homogenization in the MTZs below. Fibroblast activity and neocollagenesis take place in the MTZs, allowing for faster healing than with non-fractionated resurfacing devices. Currently, fractionated devices appear to offer the greatest hope for optimal light-based scar revision with the least downtime.

Ablative Fractional Lasers

AFLs have been reported to successfully treat moderate to severe atrophic surgical scars.[44,45] These lasers combine the increased efficacy of ablative techniques with the safety and reduced downtime associated with FP. It has been theorized that the enhanced clinical effects of AFLs are related to deeper penetration into the skin than is reached with fully ablative lasers and NAFLs, as well as prolongation of wound remodeling, to several months' duration.[14] In the treatment of atrophic surgical and traumatic scars, AFL devices have been reported to improve skin texture, pigmentation, atrophy, and overall appearance after the first session, with incremental improvements after subsequent treatments (Figure 6.4). These are usually performed every 4–6 weeks, and maximal benefit may take 3–6 months after the final session to fully appreciate.[44,46]

Optimal AFL treatment settings vary depending on the laser system being used and the individual scar characteristics. Higher fluences have been suggested to correlate with improved clinical results and patient satisfaction, whereas increased treatment densities can be associated with elevated incidence of pain, erythema, and dyspigmentation.[14,47,48] As well, higher coagulation settings are used to treat porous areas, such as the nose, while lower settings are appropriate for thin-skinned areas, such as the eyelid.

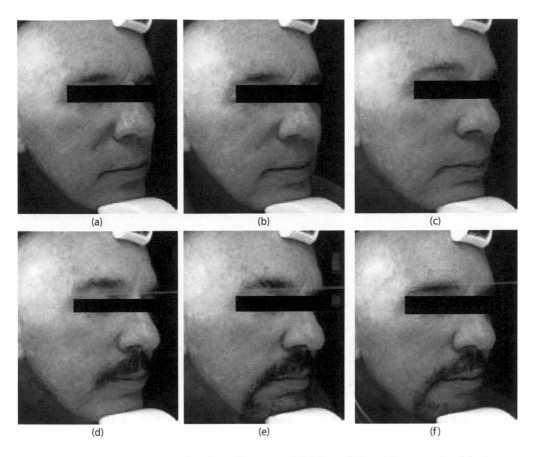

FIGURE 6.4   Scar treatment with ablative fractionated CO_2 laser (CO_2RE, Syneron-Candela, Irvine, CA) starting at 3.5 weeks after surgery. Successful revision of a surgical scar on the right medial cheek. (a) Before treatment. (b–e) During treatment. (f) After four sessions of AFL treatments. (Courtesy of Joel L. Cohen, Colorado, USA.)

Following AFL treatment, intense erythema, serosanguineous drainage, and crusting are typically seen for 5–7 days (compared to weeks to months using conventional ablative lasers or dermabrasion). Rarely, permanent hypertrophic scarring of the neck, chest, and periocular regions has been reported.[49,50] Although transient hyperpigmentation may occur, there have been no reports of persistent or permanent hypopigmentation resulting from the treatment. Thus, AFLs allow for more rapid healing and decreased likelihood of pigmentary alteration or scarring than conventional fully ablative devices.[51] Fewer side effects and quicker recovery times make AFLs a desirable therapeutic modality for scar revision.

Nonablative Fractional Lasers

NAFLs are currently the most widely studied fractional devices for scar revision.[10] These devices have shown promise in the treatment of atrophic scars, hypertrophic scars, and hypopigmented scars (Figures 6.5 and 6.6).[52] Several studies have reported significant improvement in clinical appearance, pigmentation, and thickness of surgical scars after three or four laser sessions using the 1550 nm erbium-doped fiber laser.[52,53] Some have even

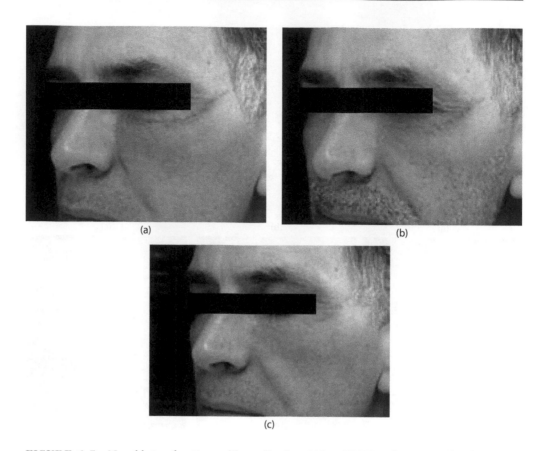

(a)

(b)

(c)

FIGURE 6.5 Nonablative fractionated laser (StarLux 500 or ICON with Lux1540 handpiece and XD Microlens, Cynosure Palomar, Westford, MA) used to treat a surgical scar. (a) Before treatment at 6.5 weeks after surgery. (b) After one treatment session using a fluence of 55 J/cm², a 15 ms pulse duration, and five passes with compression. (c) After two treatments using the same settings. Note significant improvement in scar appearance, texture, and color. (Courtesy of Joel L. Cohen, Colorado, USA.)

reported greater improvement in scar appearance after treatment with NAFL than after PDL,[53] though this would have to be confirmed with additional studies. NAFLs have been validated as a safe and effective therapeutic option for surgical scars with minimal downtime and a low incidence of adverse effects.[22,52,54,55]

Recommended settings for commonly used NAFL devices are shown in Table 6.1. A series of three to five sessions is often needed to produce perceptible clinical improvement.[56,57] Re-treatment with higher fluences can be performed at 4-week intervals until the patient is satisfied with the clinical outcome.[14] As with AFLs, higher energy settings and multiple laser passes lead to improved clinical outcomes, whereas increased density can cause greater erythema, edema, and hyperpigmentation.[58] Furthermore, NAFL resurfacing can provide an advantage over traditional nonablative laser treatments because exfoliation of the epidermis is gradual, with resultant improvement in superficial dyspigmentation.[44,59–62]

Adverse effects following NAFL treatment are typically mild and short-lived. Transient postoperative erythema, periocular edema, postinflammatory hyperpigmentation in darker skin

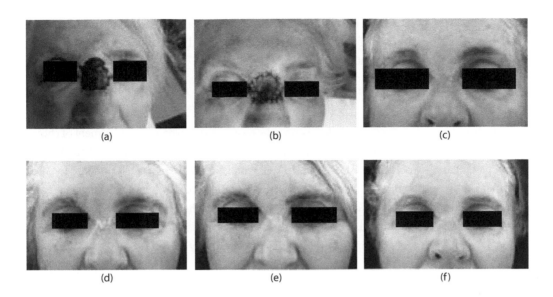

FIGURE 6.6 Nonablative fractionated laser (StarLux 500 or ICON with Lux1540 handpiece and XD Microlens, Palomar, Burlington, MA) used to treat a surgical scar. (a) Mohs surgical defect. (b) Supraclavicular skin graft to close the defect. (c) Before resurfacing at 8 months after surgery. (d, e) During treatments using a fluence of 60 J/cm² a 15 ms pulse duration, and four or five passes using compression with treatment intervals ranging from 6 weeks to 2 months for a total of five sessions. (f) Greatly improved appearance of surgical scar. (Courtesy of Joel L. Cohen, Colorado, USA.)

phototypes, and slight darkening of the skin (bronzing) during desquamation of the microscopic epidermal necrotic debris over 2–3 days may occur.[47] Acneiform and herpetic eruptions have been reported in less than 2% of patients.[14]

Thus, NAFL procedures offer an effective, less aggressive therapeutic option for patients unable or unwilling to withstand prolonged postoperative healing times associated with AFL or traditional ablative resurfacing. Additionally, a combination of NAFL and topical bimatoprost (Latisse®, Allergan, Irvine, CA), with or without a topical retinoid or topical calcineurin inhibitor, such as pimecrolimus (Elidel®, Valeant Pharmaceuticals, Laval, Quebec, Canada), has been reported to synergistically help some patients with regional hypopigmentation after ablative laser resurfacing or dermabrasion.[63]

EMERGING THERAPIES

As discussed in Chapter 7, durable fillers, such as hyaluronic acid and calcium hydroxylapatite, can be used to fill and lift postsurgical depressed scars following reconstruction of skin cancer defects.[64] Combining AFLs and injectable fillers to enhance penetration into dermal scars offers a novel therapeutic approach.[65] In addition, AFL-assisted delivery of triamcinolone acetonide has been reported to offer a safe and effective combination therapy for challenging hypertrophic scars.[66]

Finally, some newer algorithms employ a combination of laser techniques, such as PDL and AFL. Fractional radiofrequency devices, often in combination with AFLs, have also recently emerged as a possible treatment option for atrophic acne scars.[67-69] Since no literature has been published on the use of these devices for postsurgical scarring, further studies are needed to validate these potential therapeutic modalities.

CONCLUSIONS

Laser technology has evolved tremendously over the past decades to become a treatment of choice for many types of scars. Laser scar revision is optimized when a laser is selected based on the individual patient and scar characteristics. While the 585 nm PDL has been the gold standard for laser treatment of hypertrophic and keloid scars, the optimal light-based therapy for atrophic scars remains to be elucidated. AFLs are a promising modality, and their use to successfully resurface surgical scars has been validated. Although slightly less efficacious than AFLs, NAFL devices offer a great option for patients desiring a short postoperative recovery period.

REFERENCES

1. Pinheiro AL, Pozza DH, Oliveira MG, Weissmann R, Ramalho LM. Polarized light (400–2000 nm) and non-ablative laser (685 nm): A description of the wound healing process using immunohistochemical analysis. *Photomed Laser Surg* 2005;23(5):485–92.
2. Fitzpatrick RE. Treatment of inflamed hypertrophic scars using intralesional 5-FU. *Dermatol Surg* 1999;25(3):224–32.
3. Capon A, Souil E, Gauthier B, et al. Laser assisted skin closure (LASC) by using a 815-nm diode-laser system accelerates and improves wound healing. *Lasers Surg Med* 2001;28(2):168–75.
4. Kligman AM, Strauss JS. Acne; observations on dermabrasion and the anatomy of the acne pit. *Arch Dermatol* 1956;74(4):397–404.
5. Greenbaum SS, Rubin MG. Surgical pearl: The high-energy pulsed carbon dioxide laser for immediate scar resurfacing. *J Am Acad Dermatol* 1999;40(6 Pt 1):988–90.
6. Rohrer TE, Ugent SJ. Evaluating the efficacy of using a short-pulsed erbium:YAG laser for intraoperative resurfacing of surgical wounds. *Lasers Surg Med* 2002;30(2):101–5.
7. McCraw JB, McCraw JA, McMellin A, Bettencourt N. Prevention of unfavorable scars using early pulse dye laser treatments: A preliminary report. *Ann Plast Surg* 1999;42(1):7–14.
8. Ozog DM, Moy RL. A randomized split-scar study of intraoperative treatment of surgical wound edges to minimize scarring. *Arch Dermatol* 2011;147(9):1108–10.
9. Nouri K, Elsaie ML, Vejjabhinanta V, et al. Comparison of the effects of short- and long-pulse durations when using a 585-nm pulsed dye laser in the treatment of new surgical scars. *Lasers Med Sci* 2010;25(1):121–6.
10. Elsaie ML, Choudhary S. Lasers for scars: A review and evidence-based appraisal. *J Drugs Dermatol* 2010;9(11):1355–62.
11. Nouri K, Rivas MP, Stevens M, et al. Comparison of the effectiveness of the pulsed dye laser 585 nm versus 595 nm in the treatment of new surgical scars. *Lasers Med Sci* 2009;24(5):801–10.
12. Hambleton J, Shakespeare PG, Pratt BJ. The progress of hypertrophic scars monitored by ultrasound measurements of thickness. *Burns* 1992;18(4):301–7.
13. Reish RG, Eriksson E. Scar treatments: Preclinical and clinical studies. *J Am Coll Surg* 2008;206(4):719–30.
14. Sobanko JF, Alster TS. Laser treatment for improvement and minimization of facial scars. *Facial Plast Surg Clin North Am* 2011;19(3):527–42.
15. Chang CW, Ries WR. Nonoperative techniques for scar management and revision. *Facial Plast Surg* 2001;17(4):283–8.
16. Khatri KA, Mahoney DL, McCartney MJ. Laser scar revision: A review. *J Cosmet Laser Ther* 2011;13(2):54–62.
17. Alster TS. Improvement of erythematous and hypertrophic scars by the 585-nm flashlamp-pumped pulsed dye laser. *Ann Plast Surg* 1994;32(2):186–90.

18. Dierickx C, Goldman MP, Fitzpatrick RE. Laser treatment of erythematous/hypertrophic and pigmented scars in 26 patients. *Plast Reconstr Surg* 1995;95(1):84–90.
19. Fiskerstrand EJ, Svaasand LO, Volden G. Pigmentary changes after pulsed dye laser treatment in 125 northern European patients with port wine stains. *Br J Dermatol* 1998;138(3):477–9.
20. Alster T. Laser scar revision: Comparison study of 585-nm pulsed dye laser with and without intralesional corticosteroids. *Dermatol Surg* 2003;29(1):25–9.
21. Alster TS, Lewis AB, Rosenbach A. Laser scar revision: Comparison of CO_2 laser vaporization with and without simultaneous pulsed dye laser treatment. *Dermatol Surg* 1998;24(12):1299–302.
22. Tanzi EL, Alster TS. Comparison of a 1450-nm diode laser and a 1320-nm Nd:YAG laser in the treatment of atrophic facial scars: A prospective clinical and histologic study. *Dermatol Surg* 2004;30(2 Pt 1):152–7.
23. Friedman PM, Jih MH, Skover GR, Payonk GS, Kimyai-Asadi A, Geronemus RG. Treatment of atrophic facial acne scars with the 1064-nm Q-switched Nd:YAG laser: Six-month follow-up study. *Arch Dermatol* 2004;140(11):1337–41.
24. Rogachefsky AS, Hussain M, Goldberg DJ. Atrophic and a mixed pattern of acne scars improved with a 1320-nm Nd:YAG laser. *Dermatol Surg* 2003;29(9):904–8.
25. Erol OO, Gurlek A, Agaoglu G, Topcuoglu E, Oz H. Treatment of hypertrophic scars and keloids using intense pulsed light (IPL). *Aesthetic Plast Surg* 2008;32(6):902–9.
26. Bellew SG, Weiss MA, Weiss RA. Comparison of intense pulsed light to 595-nm long-pulsed pulsed dye laser for treatment of hypertrophic surgical scars: A pilot study. *J Drugs Dermatol* 2005;4(4):448–52.
27. Ortonne JP. Psoralen therapy in vitiligo. *Clin Dermatol* 1989;7(2):120–35.
28. Njoo MD, Bos JD, Westerhof W. Treatment of generalized vitiligo in children with narrow-band (TL-01) UVB radiation therapy. *J Am Acad Dermatol* 2000;42(2 Pt 1):245–53.
29. Westerhof W, Nieuweboer-Krobotova L. Treatment of vitiligo with UV-B radiation vs topical psoralen plus UV-A. *Arch Dermatol* 1997;133(12):1525–8.
30. Friedman PM, Geronemus RG. Use of the 308-nm excimer laser for postresurfacing leukoderma. *Arch Dermatol* 2001;137(6):824–5.
31. Alexiades-Armenakas MR, Bernstein LJ, Friedman PM, Geronemus RG. The safety and efficacy of the 308-nm excimer laser for pigment correction of hypopigmented scars and striae alba. *Arch Dermatol* 2004;140(8):955–60.
32. Nanni CA, Alster TS. Complications of carbon dioxide laser resurfacing. An evaluation of 500 patients. *Dermatol Surg* 1998;24(3):315–20.
33. Bernstein LJ, Kauvar AN, Grossman MC, Geronemus RG. The short- and long-term side effects of carbon dioxide laser resurfacing. *Dermatol Surg* 1997;23(7):519–25.
34. Khatri KA, Ross V, Grevelink JM, Magro CM, Anderson RR. Comparison of erbium:YAG and carbon dioxide lasers in resurfacing of facial rhytides. *Arch Dermatol* 1999;135(4):391–7.
35. Tanzi EL, Alster TS. Laser treatment of scars. *Skin Therapy Lett* 2004;9(1):4–7.
36. Lupton JR, Alster TS. Laser scar revision. *Dermatol Clin* 2002;20(1):55–65.
37. Alster TS. Cutaneous resurfacing with CO_2 and erbium: YAG lasers: Preoperative, intraoperative, and postoperative considerations. *Plast Reconstr Surg* 1999;103(2):619–32.
38. Alster TS. Clinical and histologic evaluation of six erbium:YAG lasers for cutaneous resurfacing. *Lasers Surg Med* 1999;24(2):87–92.
39. Tanzi EL, Alster TS. Treatment of atrophic facial acne scars with a dual-mode Er:YAG laser. *Dermatol Surg* 2002;28(7):551–5.
40. Fisher AA. Lasers and allergic contact dermatitis to topical antibiotics, with particular reference to bacitracin. *Cutis* 1996;58(4):252–4.
41. Alster TS, Nanni CA. Famciclovir prophylaxis of herpes simplex virus reactivation after laser skin resurfacing. *Dermatol Surg* 1999;25(3):242–6.
42. Walia S, Alster TS. Cutaneous CO_2 laser resurfacing infection rate with and without prophylactic antibiotics. *Dermatol Surg* 1999;25(11):857–61.
43. Alexiades-Armenakas MR, Dover JS, Arndt KA. The spectrum of laser skin resurfacing: Nonablative, fractional, and ablative laser resurfacing. *J Am Acad Dermatol* 2008;58(5):719–37.
44. Weiss ET, Chapas A, Brightman L, et al. Successful treatment of atrophic postoperative and traumatic scarring with carbon dioxide ablative fractional resurfacing: Quantitative volumetric scar improvement. *Arch Dermatol* 2010;146(2):133–40.
45. Cervelli V, Gentile P, Spallone D, et al. Ultrapulsed fractional CO_2 laser for the treatment of post-traumatic and pathological scars. *J Drugs Dermatol* 2010;9(11):1328–31.

46. Cohen JL. Minimizing skin cancer surgical scars using ablative fractional Er:YAG laser treatment. *J Drugs Dermatol* 2013;12(10):1171–3.

47. Graber EM, Tanzi EL, Alster TS. Side effects and complications of fractional laser photothermolysis: Experience with 961 treatments. *Dermatol Surg* 2008;34(3):301–5.

48. Metelitsa AI, Alster TS. Fractionated laser skin resurfacing treatment complications: A review. *Dermatol Surg* 2010;36(3):299–306.

49. Avram MM, Tope WD, Yu T, Szachowicz E, Nelson JS. Hypertrophic scarring of the neck following ablative fractional carbon dioxide laser resurfacing. *Lasers Surg Med* 2009;41(3):185–8.

50. Fife DJ, Fitzpatrick RE, Zachary CB. Complications of fractional CO_2 laser resurfacing: Four cases. *Lasers Surg Med* 2009;41(3):179–84.

51. Manstein D, Herron GS, Sink RK, Tanner H, Anderson RR. Fractional photothermolysis: A new concept for cutaneous remodeling using microscopic patterns of thermal injury. *Lasers Surg Med* 2004;34(5):426–38.

52. Tierney E, Mahmoud BH, Srivastava D, Ozog D, Kouba DJ. Treatment of surgical scars with nonablative fractional laser versus pulsed dye laser: A randomized controlled trial. *Dermatol Surg* 2009;35(8):1172–80.

53. Alster TS, Tanzi EL, Lazarus M. The use of fractional laser photothermolysis for the treatment of atrophic scars. *Dermatol Surg* 2007;33(3):295–9.

54. Niwa AB, Mello AP, Torezan LA, Osorio N. Fractional photothermolysis for the treatment of hypertrophic scars: Clinical experience of eight cases. *Dermatol Surg* 2009;35(5):773–7.

55. Keller R, Belda Junior W, Valente NY, Rodrigues CJ. Nonablative 1,064-nm Nd:YAG laser for treating atrophic facial acne scars: Histologic and clinical analysis. *Dermatol Surg* 2007;33(12):1470–6.

56. Vasily DB, Cerino ME, Ziselman EM, Zeina ST. Non-ablative fractional resurfacing of surgical and post-traumatic scars. *J Drugs Dermatol* 2009;8(11):998–1005.

57. Kunishige JH, Katz TM, Goldberg LH, Friedman PM. Fractional photothermolysis for the treatment of surgical scars. *Dermatol Surg* 2010;36(4):538–41.

58. Manstein D, Zurakowski D, Thongsima S, Laubach H, Chan HH. The effects of multiple passes on the epidermal thermal damage pattern in nonablative fractional resurfacing. *Lasers Surg Med* 2009;41(2):149–53.

59. Walgrave SE, Ortiz AE, MacFalls HT, et al. Evaluation of a novel fractional resurfacing device for treatment of acne scarring. *Lasers Surg Med* 2009;41(2):122–7.

60. Walgrave S, Zelickson B, Childs J, et al. Pilot investigation of the correlation between histological and clinical effects of infrared fractional resurfacing lasers. *Dermatol Surg* 2008;34(11):1443–53.

61. Gotkin RH, Sarnoff DS, Cannarozzo G, Sadick NS, Alexiades-Armenakas M. Ablative skin resurfacing with a novel microablative CO_2 laser. *J Drugs Dermatol* 2009;8(2):138–44.

62. Ortiz AE, Tremaine AM, Zachary CB. Long-term efficacy of a fractional resurfacing device. *Lasers Surg Med* 2010;42(2):168–70.

63. Massaki AB, Fabi SG, Fitzpatrick R. Repigmentation of hypopigmented scars using an erbium-doped 1,550-nm fractionated laser and topical bimatoprost. *Dermatol Surg* 2012;38(7 Pt 1):995–1001.

64. Kasper DA, Cohen JL, Saxena A, Morganroth GS. Fillers for postsurgical depressed scars after skin cancer reconstruction. *J Drugs Dermatol* 2008;7(5):486–7.

65. Sadove R. Injectable poly-L-lactic acid: A novel sculpting agent for the treatment of dermal fat atrophy after severe acne. *Aesthetic Plast Surg* 2009;33(1):113–6.

66. Waibel JS, Wulkan AJ, Shumaker PR. Treatment of hypertrophic scars using laser and laser assisted corticosteroid delivery. *Lasers Surg Med* 2013;45(3):135–40.

67. Peterson JD, Palm MD, Kiripolsky MG, Guiha IC, Goldman MP. Evaluation of the effect of fractional laser with radiofrequency and fractionated radiofrequency on the improvement of acne scars. *Dermatol Surg* 2011;37(9):1260–7.

68. Tenna S, Cogliandro A, Piombino L, Filoni A, Persichetti P. Combined use of fractional CO_2 laser and radiofrequency waves to treat acne scars: A pilot study on 15 patients. *J Cosmet Laser Ther* 2012;14(4):166–71.

69. Yeung CK, Chan NP, Shek SY, Chan HH. Evaluation of combined fractional radiofrequency and fractional laser treatment for acne scars in Asians. *Lasers Surg Med* 2012;44(8):622–30.

Chapter 7

Neuromodulators and Fillers

Suneel Chilukuri, Sailesh Konda, and Sean Bury

INTRODUCTION

Recent advances have led to the addition of neuromodulators and injectable fillers to the therapeutic armamentarium for the improvement of scars. A growing body of evidence supports their pre- and postoperative off-label use in the management of surgical scars. This chapter will review the current literature and provide a framework of treatment guidelines for this indication; evolving trends in this field will also be examined.

NEUROMODULATORS

Botulinum toxin has long been used for various neuromuscular disorders, such as cervical dystonia, spasticity, strabismus, blepharospasm, and chronic migraine.[1-3] In dermatology, plastic surgery, and otolaryngology literature, this neuromodulator also has a long history of use for cosmetic indications, such as the improvement of facial rhytids.[4,5] Its use in the amelioration of surgical scars is now also being investigated.

Biochemistry

Botulinum toxins are naturally produced by *Clostridium botulinum* bacteria, with seven distinct subtypes (A–H) recognized at this time. All possess a core neurotoxin (~150 kDa) noncovalently bound to various components that confer a protective function against acidic stomach conditions and thermal stress.[6-8] The core neurotoxin is comprised of a 50 kDa light chain, a zinc endopeptidase, attached through a disulfide bond to a 100 kDa heavy chain, which allows the toxin to bind to a neuron and to translocate across the cell membrane.

Mechanism of Action

The primary pharmacodynamic effect of current neuromodulators is chemical denervation of the treated muscle. Normal nerve signal transmission is dependent on an action potential's arriving at the presynaptic axon terminals of somatic motor nerve fibers, where a neurotransmitter, acetylcholine (Ach), is stored within presynaptic vesicles. When stimulated, a nerve terminal releases Ach, which then binds to and activates nicotinic Ach receptors on the neuromuscular junction.

Botulinum toxin decreases nerve signal transmission by preventing the release of Ach from presynaptic nerve terminals. Two types of the toxin are currently available commercially: botulinum toxin type A (BTX-A) and botulinum toxin type B (BTX-B). In the current context, only BTX-A has been studied for scar management in the published literature; hence, the current discussion will be limited to this toxin type.

BTX-A, a naturally occurring 900 kDa complex, is a protease that degrades the synaptosomal-associated protein-25 (SNAP-25) required for the fusion of presynaptic vesicles containing Ach with the presynaptic neuronal cell membrane. This mechanism effectively prevents the release of Ach, halting action potential transmission and ultimately paralyzing the postsynaptic muscle.

By selectively and temporarily paralyzing specific muscles, botulinum toxin can treat spastic disorders or fine lines and wrinkles or, more relevant to the topic at hand, release tension across wounds and scars.

Mechanism of Action in Wound Healing   The effects of BTX-A on wound healing are currently under investigation. Initial studies concentrated on its paralytic effect. Tension exerted on a wound contributes to scar elevation and the formation of hypertrophic or keloid scars.[9,10] Over time, wound tension can also lead to spread scars. Thus, BTX-A may improve final cosmesis both pre- and intraoperatively by decreasing wound tension.

Mahboub and colleagues reported successful pretreatment of 11 traumatic facial scars with onabotulinumtoxinA (Botox, Allergan, Irvine, CA) to achieve improvement following subsequent scar revision. Subjects received injections in one or two sessions until the desired muscle paralysis was achieved.[11] Flynn injected onabotulinumtoxinA intraoperatively, which also led to improved scar outcomes. Moreover, the study demonstrated that effects on *in vivo* wound healing derived primarily from decreased tension rather than from direct modulation of the wound healing response.[12]

Nonetheless, BTX-A may aid in the prevention of hypertrophic or keloid scars by reducing postsurgical inflammation. Neuromodulators have an *in vitro* inhibitory effect on the fibroblast cell cycle. Thus, fibroblasts treated with onabotulinumtoxinA spend a greater time in the quiescent (G_0) phase and less time in the actively dividing phases than control cells.[13] Lee and colleagues demonstrated that wounds exposed to onabotulinumtoxinA exhibited a smaller inflammatory cell infiltrate, fewer fibroblasts, less fibrosis, and lower transforming growth factor-β1 (TGF-β1) expression in a rat model.[14] In theory, decreased fibroblast activity should result in a smaller scar due to reduced collagen production. This was confirmed in *in vivo* rabbit ear models, in which local toxin injection inhibited the formation of hypertrophic scars through reduced fibroblast activity.[15,16]

Therapeutic Formulations, Reconstitution, and Storage

Currently, three formulations of BTX-A approved by the Food and Drug Administration (FDA) are commercially available in the United States: onabotulinumtoxinA (Botox, Allergan, Irvine, CA), incobotulinumtoxinA (Xeomin, Merz Pharma GmBH, Frankfurt, Germany), and abobotulinumtoxin A (Dysport, Medicis/Valeant, Scottsdale, AZ) (Table 7.1). Additional formulations are available around the world but are not legal for use in the United States.

While all formulations contain the 150 kDa core neurotoxin, the presence and amount of the nontoxin protein components vary. Thus, onabotulinumtoxinA and abobotulinumtoxinA are synthesized as protein complexes but differ in composition, while

TABLE 7.1   FDA-Approved Commercial Formulations of Botulinum Toxin Type A

Generic Name (Brand name)	Strain	Molecular Weight (kDa)	Units Per Vial	Storage
OnabotulinumtoxinA (Botox)	Hall	900	50/100	Refrigerated; stored 36 mo before reconstitution and 24 h after
AbobotulinumtoxinA (Dysport)	Ipsen	500–900	300	Refrigerated; stored 24 mo before reconstitution and up to 4 h after
IncobotulinumtoxinA (Xeomin)	Hall	150	50/100	Refrigerated, frozen, or kept at room temperature; stored 36 mo before reconstitution and 24 h after

incobotulinumtoxinA is formulated without any complexing proteins. These variations among products have led researchers to compare spread, efficacy, and potency. In general, there is minimal difference in clinical effect, despite the various compositions of BTX-A. Familiarity and clinical judgment often determine which product is used.

All formulations are dosed by the "unit," a measure of BTX-A that has been standardized through *in vitro* mouse assays. However, because of differences in activity, units are not equivalent among the different products. Thus, 2–4 units of abobotulinumtoxinA are required to achieve the same clinical response as 1 unit of onabotulinumtoxinA, whereas incobotulinumtoxinA and onabotulinumtoxinA are typically dosed similarly.

Prior to use, all botulinum toxins have to be reconstituted. Although preservative-free 0.9% sodium chloride (NaCl) solution is recommended as the diluent by the toxins' manufacturers, bacteriostatic NaCl solution has been found to make the injections less painful and not to affect the clinical efficacy of the product.[17] The amount of diluent may vary depending on the location of the injection and the surgeon's personal preference, but 2.5 mL of 0.9% NaCl solution is most commonly used in clinical practice. With this dilution, the resulting dose of onabotulinumtoxinA or incobotulinumtoxinA is 4 units per 0.1 mL, while that of abobotulinumtoxinA is 10 units per 0.1 mL. During reconstitution, it is recommended that the vial not be subjected to excessive movement, such as shaking, though recent studies suggest that vigorous agitation does not affect the toxin's efficacy.[18]

Once reconstituted, BTX-A has to be refrigerated and, according to the label, used within 4–24 hours (Table 7.1). However, based on published studies, the current consensus is that these toxins may be stored considerably longer.[18-20]

Common Uses in Mohs and Dermatological Surgery

Perioperative administration of neurotoxins has been shown to be safe and effective in achieving reduced scarring and optimal postsurgical results (Figure 7.1).[9,21-23] Flynn retrospectively analyzed 18 patients undergoing Mohs surgery on the face with intraoperative BTX-A or BTX-B injection and found that 17 patients reported excellent results at the 3-month follow-up.[12] Gassner and colleagues studied 31 subjects with forehead wounds. The

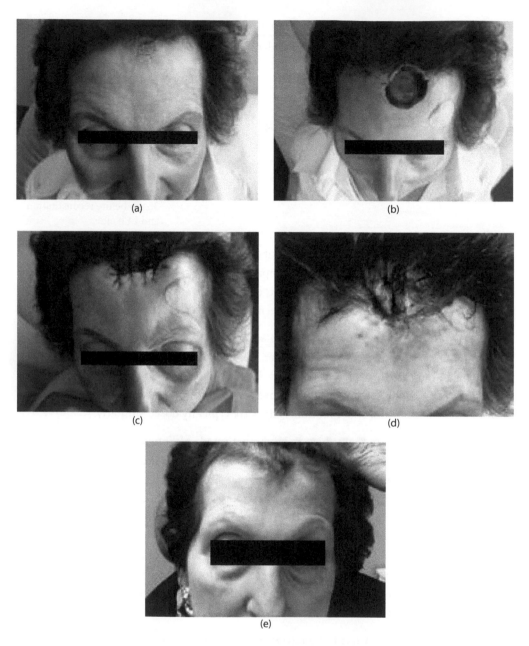

FIGURE 7.1 Botulinum toxin can be successfully used to reduce wound tension. (a) Prior to Mohs surgery for a basal cell carcinoma. Neurotoxin was injected during consultation to temporarily paralyze the frontalis muscle. (b) Defect after Mohs surgery. (c) Immediately after reconstruction. (d) At suture removal. Despite its large size, the wound did not undergo dehiscence. (e) Five months after Mohs surgery.

results demonstrated that 20–60 units of onabotulinumtoxinA administered within 24 hours of wound closure to immobilize the frontalis muscle led to enhanced healing and improved final cosmesis.[9]

Perioral and periocular surgical wounds may also benefit from perioperative BTX-A administration. Tollefson and colleagues reported safe use of intraoperative onabotulinumtoxinA injections in three infants undergoing cleft lip repair. BTX-A reduced lip tension and improved final cosmetic outcome.[23] Choi and colleagues noted excellent healing in 11 patients who were administered onabotulinumtoxinA at the time of eyelid reconstruction.[21] Furthermore, the toxin has been used intraoperatively for improved cosmetic results in blepharoplasties.[24] These findings can likely be extrapolated to Mohs and excisional wounds at these locations.

Additional Uses in Mohs Surgery   In addition to its use in scar optimization, BTX-A's anticholinergic effects have been exploited in the treatment of a postoperative complication of Mohs micrographic surgery. Several case reports have documented the use of BTX-A following parotid duct injury with resulting parotid fistula or sialocele formation.[25,26] In one such report, intraparotid administration of 23 units of onabotulinumtoxinA led to the resolution of sialoceles within 2 weeks of treatment. The patient remained asymptomatic at 6 months.[26]

Treatment Specifics

Timing of Administration   Although BTX-A is rapidly absorbed, full muscle denervation takes approximately 1 week. It is of note that, in our experience, the initial effects can be seen earlier, typically within 24–48 hours following abobotulinumtoxinA administration and within 48–96 hours with the use of onabotulinumtoxinA or incobotulinumtoxinA. Thus, for optimal effect, neuromodulators should be injected at least 1 week preoperatively. Unfortunately, not every patient can be seen in consultation prior to the day of surgery.

Clinical longevity of all neuromodulators ranges from 3 to 4 months on average. This duration, however, may be somewhat reduced in highly kinetic muscles, such as the orbicularis oris.

Dosage   Table 7.2 provides dosing recommendations for each of the three FDA-approved forms of BTX-A.[27] While these have been developed for cosmetic indications at each location, similar doses would be expected to be effective in the treatment of scars.

Technique   Prior to injecting BTX-A, a physician needs to understand the relevant neuromuscular anatomy and how previous surgical procedures can alter anatomical structures. Additionally, the surgeon should evaluate which muscles are generating significant tension vectors on the scar of interest.

Proper injection technique is crucial to achieving the desired outcome. In our clinic, we use 1 mL "No Waste" syringes (Acuderm Inc., Fort Lauderdale, FL) and a 32-gauge TSK SteriJect needle (TSK, Tochigi-Ken, Japan). Other practitioners prefer 0.5–1 mL insulin syringes that come complete with a 29-gauge needle (Becton Dickinson, Franklin Lakes, NJ). Both allow for physician precision and patient comfort.

When administering BTX-A, the needle is advanced through the skin into the underlying muscle and a predetermined aliquot is injected into each site. On average, 2–4 units of onabotulinumtoxinA or incobotulinumtoxinA or 5–10 units of abobotulinumtoxinA are placed per injection point. The total amount per muscle depends on the location and on each patient's unique muscular anatomy (Table 7.2).

TABLE 7.2   Dosage Recommendations for BTX-A Formulations

Muscle	OnabotulinumtoxinA (Botox)	AbobotulinumtoxinA (Dysport)	IncobotulinumtoxinA (Xeomin)
Frontalis	6–25 U total	20–60 U total	6–25 U total
Corrugator supercilii	8–17 U per side	20–42 U per side	8–17 U per side
Procerus	5–10 U	10–26 U	5–10 U
Orbicularis oculi	6–15 U per side	20–60 U per side	6–15 U per side
Nasalis	2–3 U	10–20 U	2–3 U
Depressor septi	2 U	5–9 U	2 U
Orbicularis oris	4–10 U per lip	10–26 U per lip	4–10 U per lip
Mentalis	2–8 U	5–20 U	2–8 U
Depressor anguli oris	3–7 U per side	5–20 U per side	3–7 U per side
Platysma	10–30 U per band	20–40 U per band	10–30 U per band

Source: Adapted from Kane M., Donofrio L., Ascher B. et al., *J Drugs Dermatol*, 9(1 Suppl), s7–22, 2010.
Note: U, units.

Injected volumes should be kept to a minimum to avoid spread of the toxin's effect. The effective spread, or diffusion, from each injection point is controversial. The average spread is 2.5–3 cm. Some researchers claim that abobotulinumtoxinA has significantly greater diffusion than onabotulinumtoxinA or incobotulinumtoxinA.[28] Other studies note that there is no distinction among the currently available neuromodulators. In our practice, we do not see a significant difference in clinical spread or longevity among these neurotoxins.

Patients should return in 1–2 weeks to be evaluated for adequate muscle paralysis. Additional toxin can be injected at that time, if deemed necessary.

Contraindications and Adverse Effects

Prior to using neurotoxins in scar management, the physician should screen the patient for contraindications. BTX-A is absolutely contraindicated in patients with neuromuscular disorders, such as peripheral motor neuropathic diseases, amyotrophic lateral sclerosis, and neuromuscular junction disorders (e.g., myasthenia gravis and Lambert-Eaton syndrome). BTX-A should be avoided in women who are pregnant, breast-feeding, or planning to become pregnant. Additionally, injections should not be administered to patients who are allergic to the neurotoxin or any ingredients in the toxin formulation, including the human albumin in all three products and lactose in Dysport.

Current medications should be thoroughly reviewed with the patient, as some may inhibit or potentiate the effect of botulinum toxin. Since BTX-A acts via a zinc-dependent mechanism, any agent that changes the tissue concentration of zinc may alter the toxin's effectiveness.[29] Some classes of such medications are angiotensin-converting enzyme (ACE) inhibitors, antibiotics, muscle relaxants, and anticholinergic agents.

De Paiva and colleagues demonstrated that the toxin's neuroparalytic activities were diminished by concurrent administration of captopril and phosphoramidon.[29]

Conversely, antibiotics such as aminoglycosides and spectinomycin may exaggerate the neuromodulating effect.[30,31] Similarly, muscle relaxants such as baclofen or tizanidine may potentiate the local effects of BTX-A. When used after toxin administration, anticholinergic medications such as amitriptyline may lead to higher incidence of such complaints as dry mouth or blurred vision.

Adverse effects encountered with BTX-A are usually transient, with the most common being pain or bruising at the injection site, headache, and blepharoptosis. To avoid ptosis, injections placed supraorbitally should be administered at least 1 cm above the bony supraorbital ridge and care should be taken to avoid the levator palpebrae superioris muscle. If ptosis occurs and is troublesome to the patient, commercially available apraclonidine eyedrops can be used for temporary reversal of the effect.[32]

A black box warning has recently been added to all neurotoxins to indicate that distant spread may result in symptoms of botulism, such as generalized weakness, dysphonia, dysarthria, trouble breathing or swallowing, loss of bladder control, and double or blurred vision. While some of these may be life-threatening, none have been associated with dermatological use of the FDA-approved formulations at the usual indicated doses.[33–35] The lethal dose of BTX-A for humans is not known but is estimated to be approximately 0.09–0.15 µg intravenously or intramuscularly for a 70 kg human.[36] It is almost impossible to reach this toxic level in typical dermatological applications. There is, however, a theoretical risk that the neuromodulator may have greater diffusion than intended when injected into inflamed skin. Therefore, caution should be used when treating patients with inflammatory cutaneous diseases (e.g., acne or psoriasis), active infections (e.g., herpes simplex or impetigo), or immunocompromised status.

INJECTABLE FILLERS

While elevated scars benefit from treatment with neuromodulators, depressed or atrophic scars may be improved with dermal fillers. The history of treating such scars with volume replacement dates back to the 1890s, when Neuber used fat grafting for facial defects.[37] More recently, the use of synthetic fillers has grown, because of their effectiveness, versatility, availability, and favorable safety profile. The ultimate goal is to find a long-lasting, nonreactive filler that provides lift, smooth irregular contours, and redistribute shadows to give an improved aesthetic result.

Biochemistry and Physical Properties of Fillers

Dermal fillers may be subdivided into autologous, biological, and synthetic types. Autologous fillers include fat and platelet-rich plasma (PRP). Biological fillers come in two main formulations—collagens and hyaluronic acids (HAs)—with further subtypes based on individual branding. Synthetic fillers include semipermanent fillers—calcium hydroxylapatite (CaHA) and poly-L-lactic acid (PLLA)—and permanent fillers—polymethylmethacrylate (PMMA) and silicone.

The physical and chemical characteristics of fillers depend on such variables as the concentration of the active ingredient, the method and percentage of cross-linking, and the composition of the carrying gel. The combination of these factors leads to unique rheological values for each filler. Two rheological variables commonly used when describing dermal fillers are complex viscosity (η^*), which relates to product flow, and elastic modulus (G'), which is a measure of the filler's ability to resist deformation, or in other words, its stiffness.[38] Thus, a filler with a high G' value has higher resistance against high tension forces and may be better suited for areas with greater muscle activity. A lower G' value signifies less stiffness, making the filler more appropriate for superficial applications.

Therapeutic Formulations

While fillers are classified according to their biochemistry, most are known by their respective brand names (Table 7.3). Additional fillers are available around the world but are not currently approved by the FDA for use in the United States.

TABLE 7.3   Dermal Fillers Currently Available in the United States

Type	Brand Name	Manufacturer	Injection Depth
Autologous			
Fat	–	–	Subcutaneous/ supraperiosteal; may also be used in dermis
PRP	–	–	Papillary and reticular dermis
Biological			
Collagen	Voluntarily withdrawn from the U.S. market		
HA	Juvéderm Ultra	Allergan	Reticular dermis
	Juvéderm Ultra Plus/XC	Allergan	Reticular dermis
	Juvéderm Voluma XC	Allergan	Subcutaneous/supraperiosteal
	Restylane and Restylane-L (contains 0.1% lidocaine)	Medicis/Valeant	Reticular dermis
	Perlane and Perlane-L (contains 0.1% lidocaine)	Medicis/Valeant	Reticular dermis
	Belotero Balance	Merz	Papillary dermis
	Prevelle Silk (contains 0.3% lidocaine)	Mentor	Reticular dermis
Synthetic			
CaHA	Radiesse	Merz	Reticular dermis/ subcutaneous
PLLA	Sculptra	Dermik/Valeant	Subcutaneous/supraperiosteal
PMMA	Artefill (contains 0.3% lidocaine)	Suneva Medical	Reticular dermis/ subcutaneous
Silicone	Various	Various	Subcutaneous/supraperiosteal

Fillers may also be subdivided into three groups based on the rheological properties described in the section "Biochemistry and Physical Properties of Fillers." Thus, CaHA (Radiesse) is in the group with the highest η^* and G' values, followed by the HA fillers Restylane and Perlane in the group with medium η^* and G' values and Juvéderm Ultra, Ultra Plus, Voluma, Belotero Balance, and Prevelle Silk in the group with low η^* and G' values.[38,39] These properties may then be exploited for specific uses, such as greater lift with higher G' values important for large-volume augmentation or reduced stiffness with lower G' values preferred for high-mobility areas, such as lips.

Common Uses in Mohs and Dermatological Surgery

Autologous Fat   Autologous fat grafting can be used to smooth contour irregularities, augment or re-create insufficient or lost volume, and treat atrophic scars. Fat grafts are harvested from donor sites, such as abdomen, thighs, or buttocks; centrifuged; and then injected into their appropriate recipient sites.

The advantages of autologous fat transfer are its ready availability and low inherent cost. Disadvantages include the labor-intensive harvesting process and varying longevity. In our experience, centrifuged fat may last only 3 to 6 months, though other investigators claim it can last up to several years after a series of injections. Improved fat graft survival may be achieved by using a "nontraumatic" blunt cannula technique, centrifugation, and immediate injection of small amounts with multiple passes.[40] Additionally, Gentile and colleagues treated 10 patients with burn and posttraumatic scars with adipose-derived stromal vascular fraction (SVF) cells and observed a 63% maintenance of restored contour after 1 year, compared with only 39% in the control group treated with centrifuged fat.[41] Finally, fat grafts containing more adipose-derived stem cells may have greater viability.[42]

Platelet-Rich Plasma   PRP has recently regained popularity as an autologous filler and fibroblast stimulator. In this process, blood is drawn from the patient and differential centrifugation is performed. PRP is then harvested from the supernatant and injected into scars. Similar to those of fat, advantages of PRP include ready availability and low cost to the practice. Disadvantages include questionable effectiveness and the need for multiple treatment sessions.

PRP contains various growth factors and cytokines and has been shown to reduce erythema and hasten wound healing.[43] In addition, PRP may be a useful adjuvant therapeutic option in the treatment of scars. In the study mentioned in the "Autologous Fat" section, Gentile and colleagues also found that scars exposed to PRP in addition to SVF had a 69% maintenance of contour after 1 year, compared with the SVF only (63%) and control (39%) groups.[44] Likewise, in a split-face trial of 14 Korean patients with acne scars, Lee and colleagues found that the combination of fractional CO_2 laser resurfacing with PRP yielded enhanced recovery with less erythema and edema, as well as improved clinical appearance at the 4-month follow-up compared to fractional resurfacing combined with normal saline for the control.[45]

These studies suggest that PRP may provide an additional benefit to wound healing either alone or as part of combination therapy. Further research on its effectiveness in surgical scars and optimal treatment parameters is warranted.

Collagen   Collagen fillers are derived from bovine, porcine, or human sources. As a result, they are immunogenic and may cause a host reaction. Two rounds of skin testing—similar to placing a purified protein derivative (PPD)—are required for many collagen fillers at least 2 weeks before therapy is initiated. Even with two negative tests, the risk of allergenicity is never completely eliminated and allergic reactions can sometimes manifest after multiple successful injections. The advantages of collagen are minimal posttreatment edema and its ability to be placed in the superficial dermis. Disadvantages again include potential immunogenicity and short longevity.[45]

Even though histological assessments have shown collagen to persist for up to 9 months,[46] most physicians report observing clinical persistence for 3–4 months. Moreover, pure collagen is currently not available in the United States; however, it is a component of PMMA filler, which will be discussed in the "Polymethylmethacrylate" section.

Hyaluronic Acid   HA is a non-sulfated glycosaminoglycan (GAG) and a natural part of the extracellular matrix, which provides a medium for collagen and elastic fibers to bind together. It also contributes to skin elasticity and hydration by attracting water, thereby increasing its volume over a thousandfold.

HA fillers may be either bacterial—derived from the fermentation of *Staphylococcus equi*—or, less commonly, avian—typically extracted from rooster combs. The latter source is less popular because of its potential allergenicity.

HA fillers with concentrations higher than 20 mg/g are considered ideal, as they displace more tissue and are thought to have a longer duration of action.[47] All HA fillers are stabilized with a single cross-linking ether bond, though the specific process and the chemical agent used for such cross-linking vary.

In the past, clinicians worried about the longevity of HA fillers. Though some injectors report duration of only 3–6 months, Richards and Rashid documented sustained volume and improved contour for 24 months after treatment of an atrophic scar.[48] Similarly, Khan et al. reported successful long-term aesthetic results after injection of Perlane, Restylane, and Juvéderm Ultra Plus into a depressed scar.[49] In our experience, results may last up to 2 years, depending on scar location and depth of product placement. Recently, Juvéderm Voluma was approved by the FDA for longevity of up to 2 years.

HA fillers are advantageous because of their low immunogenicity and their reversibility with hyaluronidase, which will be discussed in the "Adverse Effects" section. Disadvantages include a greater degree of bruising than seen with collagen fillers and more postinjection edema.[50]

Additionally, previously injected HA filler may cause difficulty in histological interpretation of a basal cell carcinoma during Mohs surgery.[51]

Calcium Hydroxylapatite   CaHA is composed of calcium and phosphate ions and is identical to the mineral portion of bones and teeth. The filler consists of synthetic CaHA microspheres suspended in an aqueous carboxymethylcellulose carrier gel. While the carrier gel dissipates within 6 months of implantation, the microspheres dissolve at a much slower rate, with clinical results persisting for as long as 12–24 months. Additionally, histological studies have demonstrated that CaHA microspheres act as scaffolding for new collagen deposition, which likely contributes to the filler's longevity.[52]

In the treatment of scars, Goldberg et al. injected CaHA into saucerized acne scars in 10 patients, with excellent improvement persisting for 12 months; however, ice pick scars did not respond to treatment.[53] Kasper et al. successfully used fillers for depressed scars from Mohs surgical reconstruction. Scars were reshaped with either CaHA or HA fillers, and all patients were extremely satisfied with the aesthetic improvement.[54]

The advantages of CaHA filler are its long duration and high G′ value, allowing for more lift, as well as low immunogenicity, though some studies have documented a risk of granuloma formation.[55,56] Inflammatory nodule formation is more common after placement into lips; thus, CaHA is contraindicated for use at this site.[57,58] Disadvantages include increased bruising due to high η^* values, resulting in the need for higher injection pressures and larger needle size. Additionally, consistent with its composition, CaHA filler shows on radiographic studies.

Poly-L-Lactic Acid   PLLA was initially approved for the treatment of HIV-associated lipodystrophy. It consists of microparticles suspended in a degradable gel. As the gel is slowly resorbed following implantation, PLLA upregulates fibroblasts to produce new collagen. This makes the filler both long-lasting, persisting for up to 2 years, and slow-acting, with final results often taking several months to manifest.[59]

PLLA is supplied as a freeze-dried preparation in sterile vials and must be reconstituted at least 2 but preferably 24 hours prior to injection to ensure adequate hydration. Reconstitution is done using 3–7 mL of sterile water, often with the addition of up to 2 mL of 1% lidocaine immediately prior to injection. A large-bore needle (26 gauge or larger) is recommended, as PLLA may clog smaller-gauge needles. Subdermal or supraperiosteal placement is required, as nodules may form if the product is injected into the dermis. Additionally, increased dilution and posttreatment massage appear to reduce the incidence of this adverse effect.[59,60]

Although not studied specifically for postsurgical scars, PLLA has been evaluated in the treatment of other types of scars, such as those from acne. Sadove used this filler to correct fat atrophy from severe acne in two patients. Three treatments were administered 4 weeks apart, with excellent results.[61] Beer injected 20 patients with moderate to severe acne or varicella scars with PLLA filler and noted significant reduction in scar size and severity over the course of seven sessions.[62] Additional studies on the use and persistence of this filler in postsurgical scars need to be performed.

The main advantages of PLLA filler are significant volumization and long duration, while its disadvantages include increased bruising due to large needle size, slow onset of neocollagenesis, and occasional nodule formation.

Polymethylmethacrylate   PMMA is composed of microspheres that provide a permanent supportive foundation for long-lasting contour correction. A skin test must be performed prior to administration, as the filler is mixed with bovine collagen, which is subsequently replaced by the patient's own connective tissue within 3 months of implantation.[63]

Though no specific studies on the use of PMMA for postsurgical scarring have been performed to date, it has been used off-label to effectively improve 96% of atrophic acne scars after subcision in one study of 14 patients.[64]

Side effects are generally mild and include injection site reactions, inflammatory and noninflammatory nodule formation, product sensitivity, infection, and, rarely, skin necrosis.[65,66] It is important to note, however, that while the permanence of PMMA is an advantage, it can also be a disadvantage, because of the inability to reverse unwanted filler without surgical extirpation.

Silicone   Injectable liquid silicone has a long history of use for soft tissue augmentation and is another viable filler option for scar correction, as it is chemically inert and inexpensive and maintains precision and permanence. Barnett and Barnett demonstrated its successful use in a case series of five patients with a history of acne scarring.[67]

Though typically related to industrial grade or adulterated product use, often by unlicensed or unskilled injectors, reports of complications, such as granuloma or nodule formation, both in the medical literature and in the lay media, have limited the use of silicone in the United States.[68] Therefore, it is not a focus of this chapter.

Treatment Specifics

Timing of Administration   Fillers can be injected at any time during the wound healing process to correct contour deformities. Of interest is a large study by Sasaki that demonstrated scar improvement with the immediate use of autologous dermal fillers following wire subcision.[69] Thus, filler injection immediately after a surgical intervention may prove beneficial.

Most commonly, however, fillers are used on the more mature scars. Although we have used fillers as early as 3 months after Mohs or excisional surgery, we typically wait months after the repair to allow for scar remodeling. In fact, atrophic scars can be treated years after initial formation.

Dosage   Filler dosage varies with the size of the defect and the substance used (Table 7.4). Experience will dictate how much product to inject. For example, Juvéderm Ultra and Ultra Plus are extremely hydrophilic, requiring approximately 4 hours to manifest the final result. Thus, scars treated with these products may need to be undercorrected. Other HA preparations, such as Restylane and Perlane, do not attract as much water. CaHA and a newer HA filler, Juvéderm Voluma, show minimal, if any, hydrophilic nature and should therefore be injected to full correction.

Technique   Physicians injecting fillers need to be familiar with the relevant neuromuscular and vascular anatomy. As with BTX-A, proper technique is crucial to achieving desired cosmetic outcomes.

TABLE 7.4   Dosages of Filler Agents Used in Published Studies on Treatment of Scars

Study	Filler	Scar Morphology	Dosage
Sasaki[68]	Autologous fat, muscle, or fascia	Facial wrinkles and scars	1–2 mm tissue strips
Lee[43]	PRP	Atrophic acne scars	0.3 mL
Richards[47]	HA	32 × 8 mm with 0.6 cm depression	Not described
Khan[48]	HA	Linear 13 cm × 2 cm with 0.8 cm depression	7 mL
Goldberg[52]	CaHA	Ice pick	0.1–0.3 mL
Beer[61]	PLLA	Depressed varicella and acne	0.2–1.5 mL (initial session); 0–1.25 mL (follow-up sessions)
Barnett[66]	Liquid silicone	Depressed acne	0.4–1.8 mL

Note: PRP, platelet-rich plasma; HA, hyaluronic acid; CaHA, calcium hydroxylapatite; PLLA, poly-L-lactic acid.

Topical anesthesia is typically sufficient for comfortable injection.[70] When filling large facial defects, the surgeon may choose to use nerve blocks.[71] The decision to provide anesthesia via the topical route or a nerve block is largely based on physician experience and preference. Additionally, all of the HA fillers available in the United States have formulations containing 0.3% lidocaine (designated as "XC" for "extra comfort" for Allergan brands and "L" for Medicis/Valeant brands), which provide incremental anesthesia with subsequent injections. Likewise, CaHA filler is shipped with a mixing kit for manual addition of lidocaine to the product, if desired. Adding it, however, changes the product's rheological properties.

Most synthetic fillers are prepackaged with a needle that is optimized for the viscosity of the product. For instance, Juvéderm Ultra flows well through the included 30-gauge needle, while the more viscous Juvéderm Ultra Plus is better delivered with a 27-gauge needle. Some HA and CaHA fillers use thin-walled needles, allowing for a larger bore size with a smaller outer gauge. In theory, this decreases skin trauma while allowing for easier extrusion of the product.

The needle is introduced into the skin according to the recommended depth of filler placement (Table 7.3). Thus, for mid-dermal and subdermal injections, the needle is guided with its bevel up at a 30- to 45-degree angle. Subdermal location can be confirmed by skin tenting when the needle is elevated; the needle should not be visible through the skin when it is properly placed. For supraperiosteal injections, the authors prefer to introduce the needle perpendicularly to the surface of the skin. Aspiration is recommended prior to deeper filler placement to avoid intra-arterial injection.

Fillers can be injected by any of five commonly used techniques (Figure 7.2).[71] Serial puncture involves injecting small, individual aliquots in sequence. This technique is recommended for superficial locations or thin skin. Retrograde linear threading entails tunneling the needle and continuously injecting the product as the needle is withdrawn; less commonly, filler may be injected in an anterograde manner, with the product injected as the

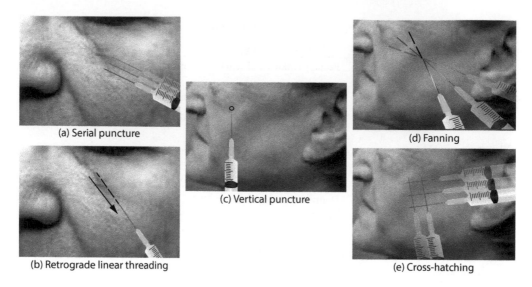

FIGURE 7.2   Filler injection techniques. (a) Serial puncture and (b) retrograde linear threading are suited for linear incisions; (c) vertical puncture is suited for small-area defects; (d) fanning and (e) cross-hatching are suited for larger-area defects.

needle is advanced. Vertical puncture may be employed to support and tense the subcutaneous connective tissue with supraperiosteal deposits. This procedure is commonly used with Juvéderm Voluma XC, the newest formulation of HA at the time of publication, though it can also be employed with other products. Fanning involves injecting multiple threads in a radial fashion without withdrawing the needle from its initial entry point. With the cross-hatching technique, multiple threads are placed perpendicularly to each other in a grid-like pattern. The last two techniques are particularly useful for augmenting larger defects.

Adverse Effects

While some adverse effects have previously been mentioned with the discussion of the individual fillers, several important general principles need to be mentioned here.

With any agent, too superficial product placement can lead to the Tyndall effect, which manifests as blue-gray discoloration due to light refraction.[72] Superficially placed HA fillers are the most common cause of iatrogenic Tyndall effect. This can be corrected by using a 30-gauge needle or a #11 blade to nick the skin in the affected areas and expressing the unwanted product. Alternatively, hyaluronidase can be used, as described later in this section.

Extreme care should be taken to avoid vascular compromise. Since post-injection edema is common with HA fillers, a large quantity placed near small vessels may lead to skin necrosis due to vascular compression. The glabella is at greatest risk, as the supratrochlear artery does not have a strong collateral circulation.[73] Another potential complication is accidental intra-arterial injection, which can result in full-thickness skin necrosis and even vision loss. Vision loss has been reported with intravascular filler injection of the angular, supraorbital, or supratrochlear artery; all of these communicate with the ophthalmic artery.[74–76] While rare, this severe complication should be suspected if a patient complains of intense pain accompanied by cutaneous blanching following injection. Application of nitroglycerin paste to induce vasodilation and administration of aspirin for anticoagulation can help reduce this sequela. Additionally, hyaluronidase should be administered if an HA product was utilized.[77]

Hyaluronidase is an enzyme that cleaves HA and can be used off-label to quickly dissolve unwanted HA filler.[78] Currently, two products are commercially available in the United States: Vitrase (Bausch & Lomb, Bridgewater, NJ) and Hylenex (Halozyme Therapeutics, San Diego, CA). Vitrase is made from purified ovine testicular hyaluronidase and is supplied at a concentration of 200 USP units/mL in 1.2 mL vials. Hylenex is a preparation of recombinant human hyaluronidase available as 1 mL vials at a concentration of 150 USP units/mL. The solution is injected directly into an HA depot in small aliquots of 7.5–15 units per site.[79] Additional hyaluronidase may be administered as needed every 10–14 days until excess HA is sufficiently dissolved.

Nodule formation is not uncommon, especially with semipermanent and permanent fillers. To lower this risk, treated areas should be firmly massaged immediately following product placement, as well as for several days posttreatment. The authors use a lotion or a gel to lubricate the skin prior to massage. This increases patient comfort and reduces erythema and bruising from this manipulation.

Additional Pearls

In evaluation of a depressed scar, bacteriostatic saline can often be used to ascertain whether a filler may improve its cosmetic appearance. This method is inexpensive and short-acting; while the saline expansion effect lasts only several minutes, it gives the patient the chance to see the potential improvement in scar contour.

We recommend HA products for the initial treatment of depressed or atrophic scars, especially for a beginning injector. The advantage of these agents is their reversibility with hyaluronidase. In addition, there are multiple types of HA fillers, each with unique clinical properties. For example, we find that Juvéderm Voluma, currently the only FDA-approved filler for the mid-face, provides the greatest amount of lift when a scar is located over a bony prominence. On the other hand, as previously discussed, Perlane and Restylane have excellent stiffness (G′) and can be used in the mid-cheek with the cross-hatch method. Large depressed scars may be corrected with Juvéderm Ultra and Ultra Plus, because of these fillers' hydrophilic nature. When either of these two products is placed with the fanning technique, significant volume restoration can be obtained (Figure 7.3).

Once the HA filler is resorbed, a longer-lasting product, such as CaHA, PMMA, or PLLA, may be considered. For small defects less than 3 cm long, we prefer PMMA if the patient has a negative skin test. For larger defects, we find great success with the PLLA filler.

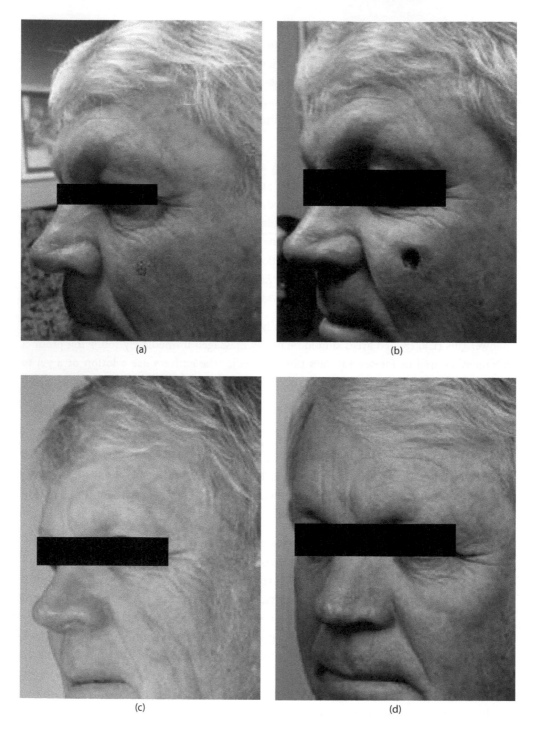

FIGURE 7.3   Fillers may aid in the re-creation of smooth contour. (a) Before Mohs surgery for a squamous cell carcinoma.(b) Defect after Mohs surgery. (c) Eight months after surgery, the patient is bothered by the indentation at the surgical site. Juvéderm Ultra Plus and Voluma fillers were used for volumization. (d) One month after filler injection. Patient demonstrates excellent improvement in scar contour.

CONCLUSIONS

Neuromodulators and fillers have become important additions to the field of scar management and should be considered in the appropriate clinical settings. Neuromodulators demonstrate promise in the prevention and treatment of hypertrophic and keloid scars, whereas fillers have been shown to improve depressed scars. Additional studies are needed to further evaluate these products in the treatment of postsurgical scars.

REFERENCES

1. Hallett M, Albanese A, Dressler D, et al. Evidence-based review and assessment of botulinum neurotoxin for the treatment of movement disorders. *Toxicon* 2013;67:94–114.
2. Czyz CN, Burns JA, Petrie TP, Watkins JR, Cahill KV, Foster JA. Long-term botulinum toxin treatment of benign essential blepharospasm, hemifacial spasm, and Meige syndrome. *Am J Ophthalmol* 2013;156(1):173–7.
3. Jackson JL, Kuriyama A, Hayashino Y. Botulinum toxin A for prophylactic treatment of migraine and tension headaches in adults: A meta-analysis. *JAMA* 2012;307(16):1736–45.
4. Carruthers JD, Carruthers JA. Treatment of glabellar frown lines with *C. botulinum*-A exotoxin. *J Dermatol Surg Oncol* 1992;18(1):17–21.
5. Blitzer A, Brin MF, Keen MS, Aviv JE. Botulinum toxin for the treatment of hyperfunctional lines of the face. *Arch Otolaryngol Head Neck Surg* 1993;119(9):1018–22.
6. Chen F, Kuziemko GM, Stevens RC. Biophysical characterization of the stability of the 150-kilodalton botulinum toxin, the nontoxic component, and the 900-kilodalton botulinum toxin complex species. *Infect Immun* 1998;66(6):2420–5.
7. Ohishi I, Sugii S, Sakaguchi G. Oral toxicities of *Clostridium botulinum* toxins in response to molecular size. *Infect Immun* 1977;16(1):107–9.
8. Sugii S, Ohishi I, Sakaguchi G. Intestinal absorption of botulinum toxins of different molecular sizes in rats. *Infect Immun* 1977;17(3):491–6.
9. Gassner HG, Brissett AE, Otley CC, et al. Botulinum toxin to improve facial wound healing: A prospective, blinded, placebo-controlled study. *Mayo Clin Proc* 2006;81(8):1023–8.
10. Freshwater MF. Botulinum toxin for scars: Can it work, does it work, is it worth it? *J Plast Reconstr Aesthet Surg* 2013;66(3):e92–e93.
11. Mahboub T, Sobhi A, Habashi H. Optimization of presurgical treatment with botulinum toxin in facial scar management. *Egypt J Plast Reconstr Surg* 2006;30:81–6.
12. Flynn TC. Use of intraoperative botulinum toxin in facial reconstruction. *Dermatol Surg* 2009;35(2):182–8.
13. Zhibo X, Miaobo Z. Botulinum toxin type A affects cell cycle distribution of fibroblasts derived from hypertrophic scar. *J Plast Reconstr Aesthet Surg* 2008;61(9):1128–9.
14. Lee BJ, Jeong JH, Wang SG, Lee JC, Goh EK, Kim HW. Effect of botulinum toxin type A on a rat surgical wound model. *Clin Exp Otorhinolaryngol* 2009;2(1):20–7.
15. Wang L, Tai NZ, Fan ZH. Effect of botulinum toxin type A injection on hypertrophic scar in rabbit ear model. [In Chinese.] *Zhonghua Zheng Xing Wai Ke Za Zhi* 2009;25(4):284–7.
16. Xiao Z, Qu G. Effects of Botulinum toxin type A on collagen deposition in hypertrophic scars. *Molecules* 2012;17(2):2169–77.
17. Allen SB, Goldenberg NA. Pain difference associated with injection of abobotulinumtoxinA reconstituted with preserved saline and preservative-free saline: A prospective, randomized, side-by-side, double-blind study. *Dermatol Surg* 2012;38(6):867–70.
18. Shome D, Nair AG, Kapoor R, Jain V. Botulinum toxin A: Is it really that fragile a molecule? *Dermatol Surg* 2010;36 Suppl 4:2106–10.
19. Liu A, Carruthers A, Cohen JL, et al. Recommendations and current practices for the reconstitution and storage of botulinum toxin type A. *J Am Acad Dermatol* 2012 Sep;67(3):373–8.
20. Trindade De Almeida AR, Secco LC, Carruthers A. Handling botulinum toxins: An updated literature review. *Dermatol Surg* 2011;37(11):1553–65.

21. Choi JC, Lucarelli MJ, Shore JW. Use of botulinum A toxin in patients at risk of wound complications following eyelid reconstruction. *Ophthal Plast Reconstr Surg* 1997;13 (4): 259–64.
22. Zimbler MS, Nassif PS. Adjunctive applications for botulinum toxin in facial aesthetic surgery. *Facial Plast Surg Clin North Am* 2003;11 (4):477–82.
23. Tollefson TT, Senders CM, Sykes JM, Byorth PJ. Botulinum toxin to improve results in cleft lip repair. *Arch Facial Plast Surg* 2006;8(3):221–2.
24. Guerrissi JO. Intraoperative injection of botulinum toxin A into the orbicularis oculi muscle for the treatment of crow's feet. *Plast Reconstr Surg* 2003;112 Suppl 5:161S–163S.
25. Hatzis GP, Finn R. Using botox to treat a Mohs defect repair complicated by a parotid fistula. *J Oral Maxillofac Surg* 2007;65(11):2357–60.
26. Krishnan RS, Clark DP, Donnelly HB. The use of botulinum toxin in the treatment of a parotid duct injury during Mohs surgery and review of management options. *Dermatol Surg* 2009;35(6):941–7.
27. Kane M, Donofrio L, Ascher B, et al. Expanding the use of neurotoxins in facial aesthetics: A consensus panel's assessment and recommendations. *J Drugs Dermatol* 2010;9 Suppl 1:s7–22.
28. Kerscher M, Roll S, Becker A, Wigger-Alberti W. Comparison of the spread of three botulinum toxin type A preparations. *Arch Dermatol Res* 2012;304:155–61.
29. de Paiva A, Ashton AC, Foran P, Schiavo G, Montecucco C, Dolly JO. Botulinum A like type B and tetanus toxins fulfils criteria for being a zinc-dependent protease. *J Neurochem* 1993;61:2338–41.
30. Santos JI, Swensen P, Glasgow LA. Potentiation of *Clostridium botulinum* toxin by aminoglycoside antibiotics: Clinical and laboratory observations. *Pediatrics* 1981;68(1):50–4.
31. Vartanian AJ, Dayan SH. Complications of botulinum toxin A use in facial rejuvenation. *Facial Plast Surg Clin North Am* 2005;13(1):1–10.
32. Scheinfeld N. The use of apraclonidine eyedrops to treat ptosis after the administration of botulinum toxin to the upper face. *Dermatol Online J* 2005;11(1):9.
33. Bakheit AM, Ward CD, McLellan DL. Generalised botulism-like syndrome after intramuscular injections of botulinum toxin type A: A report of two cases. *J Neurol Neurosurg Psychiatry* 1997;62(2):198.
34. Coban A, Matur Z, Hanagasi HA, Parman Y. Iatrogenic botulism after botulinum toxin type A injections. *Clin Neuropharmacol* 2010;33(3):158–60.
35. Chertow DS, Tan ET, Maslanka SE, et al. Botulism in 4 adults following cosmetic injections with an unlicensed, highly concentrated botulinum preparation. *JAMA* 2006;296(20):2476–9.
36. Arnon SS, Schechter R, Inglesby TV, et al. Botulinum toxin as a biological weapon: Medical and public health management. *JAMA* 2001;285(8):1059–70.
37. Neuber F. Fettransplantation. *Chir Kongr Verhandl Dsch Gesellch Chir* 1895;22:66.
38. Sundaram H, Voigts B, Beer K, Meland M. Comparison of the rheological properties of viscosity and elasticity in two categories of soft tissue fillers: Calcium hydroxylapatite and hyaluronic acid. *Dermatol Surg* 2010;36 Suppl 4:1859–65.
39. Gamboa GM, Ross WA. Autologous fat transfer in aesthetic facial recontouring. *Ann Plast Surg* 2013;70(5):513–6.
40. Gentile P, De Angelis B, Pasin M, et al. Adipose-derived stromal vascular fraction cells and platelet-rich plasma: Basic and clinical evaluation for cell-based therapies in patients with scars on the face. *J Craniofac Surg* 2014;25(1):267–72.
41. Pu LLQ. Towards more rationalized approach to autologous fat grafting. *J Plast Reconstr Aesthet Surg* 2012;65(4):413–9.
42. Na JI, Choi JW, Choi HR, et al. Rapid healing and reduced erythema after ablative fractional carbon dioxide laser resurfacing combined with the application of autologous platelet-rich plasma. *Dermatol Surg* 2011;37(4):463–8.
43. Lee JW, Kim BJ, Kim MN, Mun SK. The efficacy of autologous platelet rich plasma combined with ablative carbon dioxide fractional resurfacing for acne scars: A simultaneous split-face trial. *Dermatol Surg* 2011;37(7):931–8.
44. Narins RS, Bowman PH. Injectable skin fillers. *Clin Plast Surg* 2005;32(2):151–62.
45. Cockerham K, Hsu VJ. Collagen-based dermal fillers: Past, present, future. *Facial Plast Surg* 2009;25(2):106–13.
46. Gold MH. Use of hyaluronic acid fillers for the treatment of the aging face. *Clin Interv Aging* 2007;2(3):369–76.
47. Richards KN, Rashid RM. Twenty-four-month persistence of hyaluronic acid filler for an atrophic scar. *J Cosmet Dermatol* 2011;10(4):311–2.

48. Khan F, Richards K, Rashid RM. Hyaluronic acid filler for a depressed scar. *Dermatol Online J* 2012;18(5):15.

49. Homicz MR, Watson D. Review of injectable materials for soft tissue augmentation. *Facial Plast Surg* 2004;20(1):21–9.

50. Bennett R, Taher M. Restylane persistent for 23 months found during Mohs micrographic surgery: A source of confusion with hyaluronic acid surrounding basal cell carcinoma. *Dermatol Surg* 2005;31(10):1366–9.

51. Berlin AL, Hussain M, Goldberg DJ. Calcium hydroxylapatite filler for facial rejuvenation: A histologic and immunohistochemical analysis. *Dermatol Surg* 2008;34 Suppl 1:S64–S67.

52. Goldberg DJ, Amin S, Hussain M. Acne scar correction using calcium hydroxylapatite in a carrier-based gel. *J Cosmet Laser Ther* 2006;8(3):134–6.

53. Kasper DA, Cohen JL, Saxena A, Morganroth GS. Fillers for postsurgical depressed scars after skin cancer reconstruction. *J Drugs Dermatol* 2008;7(5):486–7.

54. Coleman KM, Voigts R, DeVore DP, Termin P, Coleman WP 3rd. Neocollagenesis after injection of calcium hydroxylapatite composition in a canine model. *Dermatol Surg* 2008;34 Suppl 1:S53–S55.

55. Moulonguet I, Arnaud E, Bui P, Plantier F. Foreign body reaction to Radiesse: 2 cases. *Am J Dermatopathol* 2013;35(3):e37–e40.

56. Sankar V, McGuff HS. Foreign body reaction to calcium hydroxylapatite after lip augmentation. *J Am Dent Assoc* 2007;138(8):1093–6.

57. Tzikas TL. A 52-month summary of results using calcium hydroxylapatite for facial soft tissue augmentation. *Dermatol Surg* 2008;34 Suppl 1:S9–S15.

58. Sadick NS. Poly-L-lactic acid: A perspective from my practice. *J Cosmet Dermatol* 2008;7(1):55–60.

59. Rossner F, Rossner M, Hartmann V, Erdmann R, Wiest LG, Rzany B. Decrease of reported adverse events to injectable polylactic acid after recommending an increased dilution: 8-year results from the Injectable Filler Safety study. *J Cosmet Dermatol* 2009;8(1):14–8.

60. Sadove R. Injectable poly-L-lactic acid: A novel sculpting agent for the treatment of dermal fat atrophy after severe acne. *Aesthetic Plast Surg* 2009;33(1):113–6.

61. Beer K. A single-center, open-label study on the use of injectable poly-L-lactic acid for the treatment of moderate to severe scarring from acne or varicella. *Dermatol Surg* 2007;33 Suppl 2:S159–S167.

62. Lemperle G, Knapp TR, Sadick NS, Lemperle SM. Artefill permanent injectable for soft tissue augmentation: I. Mechanism of action and injection techniques. *Aesthetic Plast Surg* 2010;34(3):264–72.

63. Epstein RE, Spencer JM. Correction of atrophic scars with Artefill: An open-label pilot study. *J Drugs Dermatol* 2010;9(9):1062–4.

64. Cohen SR, Berner CF, Busso M, et al. Artefill: A long-lasting injectable wrinkle filler material—summary of the U.S. Food and Drug Administration trials and a progress report on 4- to 5-year outcomes. *Plast Reconstr Surg* 2006;118 Suppl 3:64S–76S.

65. Cohen JL. Understanding, avoiding, and managing dermal filler complications. *Dermatol Surg* 2008;34 Suppl 1:S92–S99.

66. Barnett JG, Barnett CR. Treatment of acne scars with liquid silicone injections: 30-year perspective. *Dermatol Surg* 2005;31(11 Pt 2):1542–9.

67. Narins RS, Beer K. Liquid injectable silicone: A review of its history, immunology, technical considerations, complications, and potential. *Plast Reconstr Surg* 2006;118 Suppl 3:77S–84S.

68. Sasaki GH. Comparison of results of wire subcision performed alone, with fills, and/or with adjacent surgical procedures. *Aesthet Surg J* 2008;28(6):619–26.

69. Sobanko JF, Miller CJ, Alster TS. Topical anesthetics for dermatologic procedures: A review. *Dermatol Surg* 2012;38(5):709–21.

70. Countryman NB, Hanke CW. Practical review of peripheral nerve blocks in dermatologic surgery of the face. *Curr Derm Rep* 2012;1:49–54.

71. Sherman RN. Avoiding dermal filler complications. *Clin Dermatol* 2009;27:S23–S32.

72. Glaich AS, Cohen JL, Goldberg LH. Injection necrosis of the glabella: Protocol for prevention and treatment after use of dermal fillers. *Dermatol Surg* 2006;32(2):276–81.

73. Kim EG, Eom TK, Kang SJ. Severe visual loss and cerebral infarction after injection of hyaluronic acid gel. *J Craniofac Surg* 2014;25(2):684–6.

74. Kim YJ, Choi KS. Bilateral blindness after filler injection. *Plast Reconstr Surg* 2013;131(2):298e–299e.

75. Roberts SA, Arthurs BP. Severe visual loss and orbital infarction following periorbital aesthetic poly-(L)-lactic acid (PLLA) injection. *Ophthal Plast Reconstr Surg* 2012;28(3):e68–e70.

76. Kim DW, Yoon ES, Ji YH, Park SH, Lee BI, Dhong ES. Vascular complications of hyaluronic acid fillers and the role of hyaluronidase in management. *J Plast Reconstr Aesthet Surg* 2011;64(12):1590–5.
77. Vartanian AJ, Frankel AS, Rubin MG. Injected hyaluronidase reduces Restylane-mediated cutaneous augmentation. *Arch Facial Plast Surg* 2005;7(4):231–7.
78. Rzany B, Becker-Wegerich P, Bachmann F, Erdmann R, Wollina U. Hyaluronidase in the correction of hyaluronic acid-based fillers: A review and a recommendation for use. *J Cosmet Dermatol* 2009;8(4):317–23.
79. Kablik J, Monheit GD, Yu L, Chang G, Gershkovich J. Comparative physical properties of hyaluronic acid dermal fillers. *Dermatol Surg* 2009;35 Suppl 1:302–12.

Chapter 8

Topical and Intralesional Therapies

Ali M. Rkein and David M. Ozog

INTRODUCTION

This concluding chapter will review the topical and intralesional treatments available for scar modulation. While many of these therapies are used for the improvement of elevated postsurgical scars, including keloids and hypertrophic scars (Figures 8.1 through 8.4), other characteristics, such as scar firmness and erythema, can also be affected by these modalities. In addition to some time-honored and well-established interventions, the chapter will also evaluate the evidence for and against some commonly used agents and present several emerging therapies.

DRESSINGS
Pressure Therapy

Pressure dressings have been commonly used in burn and hypertrophic scar management since the 1960s. The exact mechanism of action is not known, but it is believed that pressure thins the dermis and decreases edema and blood flow, producing a hypoxic environment. This may result in fibroblast degeneration and decreased collagen synthesis.[1] However, alternative mechanisms have also been suggested. Pressure therapy appears to increase the expression of prostaglandin E_2 and to inhibit the expression of transforming growth factor-β1 (TGF-β1). These changes result in increased expression of collagenases and inhibition of differentiation of fibroblasts into myofibroblasts, respectively.[2,3]

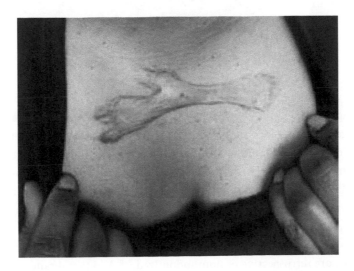

FIGURE 8.1 Partially treated keloid on chest.

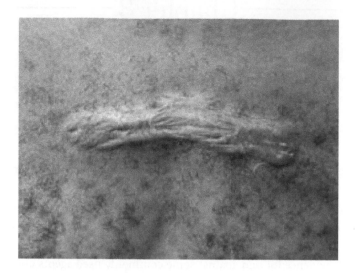

FIGURE 8.2   Untreated keloid on chest.

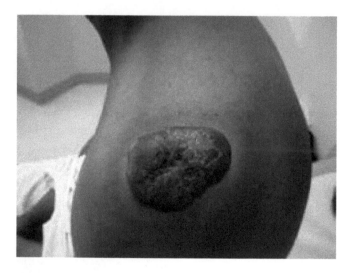

FIGURE 8.3   Untreated keloid on left shoulder.

There are many different methods for applying pressure to scars. These include elastic bandages, compression gloves for the hands, and custom-fitted compression garments. Custom-fitted garments are used for more difficult areas, including the face, neck, and trunk. They are supplied by many manufacturers and include such brands as Jobst (BSN Medical, Hamburg, Germany) and Bio-Form (Bio Concepts, Phoenix, AZ). The recommended pressure is 25 mm Hg for 6–12 months, although lower pressures may also be effective.[4] One of the main drawbacks of compression garments is the fact that they can be uncomfortable and relatively costly, leading to a lack of compliance by patients.[5] Though many studies support the efficacy of compression therapy, especially in improving or preventing the recurrence of ear keloids, most are retrospective or nonrandomized.[6-9] Additional randomized controlled studies, especially in the setting of postsurgical keloids and hypertrophic scars, are needed.

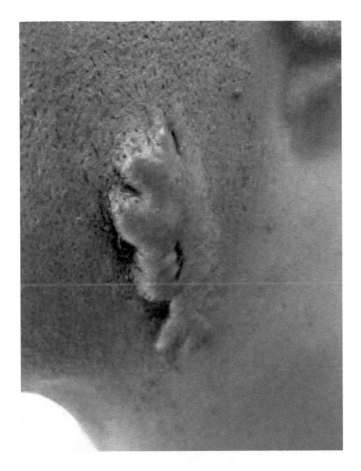

FIGURE 8.4   Untreated keloid on left cheek.

In clinical practice, the use of pressure treatment for scar reduction typically serves as an adjunct to other methods.

Adhesive Microporous Hypoallergenic Paper Tape

Paper tape, such as Micropore Medical Tape (3M, St Paul, MN), is thought to work similarly to pressure dressings but also to provide a hydrating environment (Figure 8.5). Its exact mechanism of action is not well understood. In a study involving 64 excisions on the neck, elbow, wrist, chest, and breast, paper tape was found to be helpful in preventing hypertrophic scarring when applied for a minimum of 2 months beginning 2 weeks after surgery.[10] However, a meta-analysis examining this product found that its efficacy was inferior to that of products such as silicone gel.[11]

Silicone Dressings

Silicone is a synthetic polymer with silicon and oxygen serving as its backbone. Silicone products are available as impregnated elastic sheets, gel sheets, and topical creams and gels. Silicone dressings have many advantages over other dressings: they are relatively inexpensive, painless, well tolerated, and easy to use.

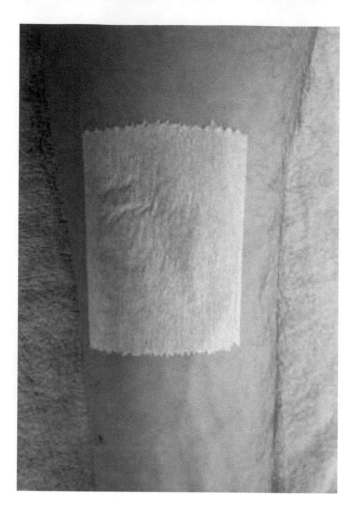

FIGURE 8.5   Example of adhesive microporous hypoallergenic paper tape on forearm.

The exact mechanism of action of silicone dressings is not well understood, but they are believed to decrease scar formation through wound hydration, an increase in static charge, and modulation of growth factors.[12,13] Silicone gel has been shown to increase basic fibroblast growth factor (bFGF) levels in normal and fetal fibroblasts and to decrease other pro-fibrotic cytokines, such as TGF-β2 and interleukin-1 (IL-1).[14,15]

A Cochrane Database Review examined the ability of silicone gel sheets to prevent and treat hypertrophic and keloid scars.[16] Prevention studies appeared to suggest that silicone gel sheets reduced the incidence of hypertrophic scars in susceptible patients, while treatment studies demonstrated a statistically significant reduction in scar length, width, and thickness, as well as improvement in scar color. However, the review noted that most studies were poorly designed and included significant bias; it concluded that the evidence for the beneficial effects of silicone gel sheets on scarring was weak and that a more rigorous evaluation was warranted.

In a study comparing the effects of silicone gel dressings, pressure therapy, and combination therapy on hypertrophic scars, silicone gel sheets were found to be more effective in reducing pain and pruritus, while pressure therapy demonstrated more improvement in scar thickness. Combination therapy was shown to lead to the most significant reduction in scar thickness.[17]

Though numerous brands of silicone gel sheets are available on the market, studies comparing their effectiveness are few. A study of two commonly used dressings, Cica-Care (Smith & Nephew, London, UK) and Silastic Gel Sheeting (Dow Corning, Midland, MI), found no difference in efficacy or safety but noted that patients thought Cica-Care gel sheets to be more adhesive and comfortable.[18] Silicone gel sheets are applied after complete reepithelization and should be used for at least 12 hours a day for a total of 2–3 months. Few adverse effects have been noted, the most common being skin maceration.

TOPICAL AGENTS
Topical Onion Extract

Onion (*Allium cepa*) extract is available in a topical over-the-counter gel (Mederma, Merz Pharma, Frankfurt, Germany) and is marketed for the treatment of hypertrophic scars. The mechanism of action is not well understood, but it is thought to possess anti-inflammatory and bacteriostatic properties.[19]

In a rabbit ear model of hypertrophic scarring, there was a significant improvement in dermal collagen organization in onion extract–treated scars compared to those in the untreated controls.[20] However, a prospective randomized double-blinded study found that a topical onion extract did not improve cosmetic appearance, erythema, or hypertrophy in new surgical scars more than petrolatum jelly did.[21] In fact, an earlier pilot study demonstrated an improvement in post-Mohs surgical scar erythema with petrolatum jelly but not with the onion extract.[22] Thus, although popular, onion extract preparations are not recommended.

Vitamin Derivatives

Vitamin E   Vitamin E is a group of eight fat-soluble compounds that include both tocopherols and tocotrienols. These compounds are identified by the prefixes α-, β-, γ-, and δ-. Different forms of vitamin E have different biological effects. For example, α-tocopherol is an antioxidant agent that protects cell membranes from oxidation through the glutathione peroxidase pathway.

Vitamin E is anecdotally thought to improve healing and decrease scar formation. This may be due to its ability to inhibit fibroblasts and keratinocytes; stimulate bFGF, thereby downregulating collagen production; and reduce the damaging effects of reactive oxygen species.[23] However, a study on the effects of topical vitamin E in patients undergoing Mohs surgery found that it either did not improve or actually worsened the cosmetic appearance of wounds compared to a standard emollient ointment. Furthermore, 33% of study subjects developed contact dermatitis to vitamin E.[24] Several other prospective studies have demonstrated similar findings,[25] so while it is popular, topical vitamin E is not recommended after cutaneous surgery.

Vitamin D   Vitamin D is a designation for a group of fat-soluble steroid hormones that function to maintain normal blood levels of calcium and phosphorus. The two forms of vitamin D that are important in humans are ergocalciferol (vitamin D_2) and cholecalciferol (vitamin D_3). Vitamin D_2 is synthesized by plants, while vitamin D_3 is synthesized by humans in the skin when it is exposed to ultraviolet B (UVB) light. Several synthetic vitamin D derivatives are currently available for the treatment of psoriasis, such as a calcipotriene cream (Dovonex®, Warner Chilcott, Dublin, Ireland).

The mechanism of action is not well understood, but vitamin D is believed to induce keratinocyte terminal differentiation, decrease keratinocyte proliferation, and decrease Langerhans cell function.[26–28] However, a recent randomized controlled study evaluated topical calcipotriene for prevention of hypertrophic scars after bilateral reduction mammoplasty and found no improvement in scar appearance after 3 months of application.[29] Thus, topical vitamin D derivatives are not recommended as postsurgical scar therapy at this time.

Retinoids   Retinoids are signaling molecules that influence the development of cells. All-trans retinoic acid (RA) and other active retinoids are generated from vitamin A (retinol) and induce differentiation primarily by binding to transcription factors in the nucleus. Topical retinoids are thought to enhance wound healing through the induction of neovascularization and the formation of collagen.[30]

Multiple studies have examined the effects of retinoids on wound healing, and the results have been conflicting. In a randomized controlled study, Otley et al. evaluated high-tension excisional wounds and full-thickness skin grafts treated perioperatively with tretinoin in a porcine model. The study concluded that topical tretinoin did not enhance the healing of excisional wounds and was detrimental to the survival of full-thickness skin grafts.[31] Gunes Bilgili et al. examined the effects of oral and topical retinoids on secondary wound healing in a rat model and concluded that both can delay secondary wound healing, epithelialization, and angiogenesis.[32] Abdelmalek and Spencer reviewed the evidence for the role of topical and systemic retinoids in wound healing. They concluded that pretreatment with retinoids likely promotes healing after facial resurfacing and that, while results are mixed regarding their effect on fresh and healing wounds, the majority of the evidence favored their use in this setting.[33] Because the role of retinoids in wound healing is still controversial, however, they are not recommended at this time.

Imiquimod

Topical imiquimod cream is an immune response modifier, which up-regulates the production of interferon-α (IFN-α), a proinflammatory cytokine that increases collagen breakdown. It has also been shown to induce other tumor necrosis factors and interleukins.[34]

The use of imiquimod for the treatment of scars has yielded mixed results. In one study, 5% imiquimod cream was applied nightly for 8 weeks following surgical removal of 13 keloids from 12 patients. At the 24-week follow-up, none of the keloids had recurred.[35] However, not all investigations have demonstrated such promising results. In a different study, nine patients applied imiquimod 5% cream for 8 weeks after surgical excision of truncal keloids. Keloids recurred in eight patients, while one patient was lost to follow-up.[36] Another study found that after excision of three presternal keloids, all of them recurred within 4 weeks of stopping the medication.[37] Thus, the role of imiquimod in the treatment and prevention of hypertrophic scars and keloids needs further investigation.

Herbal/Alternative Medicines

Increasingly, patients are turning to herbal medications for various maladies, including the treatment of scars. While anecdotal evidence and a few case reports suggest beneficial effects of some herbs for this indication, no controlled clinical trials are available at this time to examine their safety and efficacy.

Spathodea campanulata Beauv, also known as the African tulip tree, is a deciduous flowering tree native to sub-Saharan Africa and used in traditional African herbal medicine for the treatment of ulcers, filariasis, gonorrhea, diarrhea, and fever. One study demonstrated improved healing after a burn using its bark extract in a mouse model.[38]

Centella asiatica, also known as centella, is a perennial plant that grows around the Indian Ocean and is used by natives to treat small wounds, superficial burns, and hypertrophic scars. In one study, a hydrogel formulated from its extract showed significantly reduced healing time in cutaneous wounds in rats.[39]

Anogeissus latifolia, also known as axlewood, is a medium-sized plant native to India, Nepal, Myanmar, and Sri Lanka. It is used by natives to treat dysentery, snakebites, leprosy, and cutaneous wounds and ulcers. Ethanolic extract of *A. latifolia* bark was found to accelerate wound healing in rats and to increase wound tensile strength.[40] While these case reports are interesting, more clinical studies are needed to further investigate the role of herbal medications in wound healing.

INTRALESIONAL AGENTS

Corticosteroids

Intralesional corticosteroids are commonly used in the management of hypertrophic scars. When used alone, studies show their efficacy to range between 50 and 100%.[41] The mechanisms of action are thought to be primarily inhibition of the inflammatory response, promotion of collagen degeneration, and inhibition of fibroblast growth. Corticosteroids have been shown to suppress the expression of TGF-β1 and TGF-β2 but not that of TGF-β3; it is of note that scarless (fetal-like) wound healing is associated with decreased TGF-β1 and TGF-β2 activity and with increased TGF-β3 activity.[42] In addition, corticosteroids decrease the levels of α1-antitrypsin and α2-macroglobulin, both of which are collagenase inhibitors.[43] A study using three-dimensional imaging to calculate the volume of keloids and to measure their response to intralesional steroids found that the majority of patients had greater than 50% improvement within 8 weeks of starting therapy.[44]

Triamcinolone acetonide (Kenalog®, Bristol-Myers Squibb, New York, NY) is commonly used in concentrations ranging from 10 to 20 mg/mL with injections repeated every 4–6 weeks; concentrations up to 40 mg/mL can be used for bulky and resistant lesions.[45] At the authors' home institution, excellent results have been attained by injecting excised earlobe and facial keloids with triamcinolone acetonide 40 mg/mL on the day of surgery and repeating the injections at weeks 1, 2, 4, 6, 10, and 14 (Figures 8.6 through 8.8).

Up to 63% of patients can experience adverse effects with intralesional steroids, including hypopigmentation, dermal atrophy, telangiectasia, and widening of the scar (Figure 8.9).

Care must be taken when injecting into keloids: steroids must be injected intradermally, since injecting too superficially can cause irreversible epidermal atrophy, while injecting too deeply can cause fat atrophy. In addition, due to their firmness, keloids often require high injection pressure, which may result in backsplash or spraying through skin pores. Personal protective equipment, such as goggles for patients and surgical personnel, is important in this setting. Alternatively, light cryotherapy or a vascular-specific laser can be used to pretreat the lesion and to induce temporary edema, which facilitates the injection.

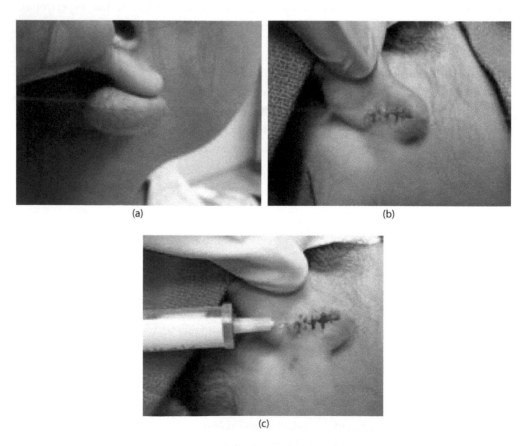

(a)

(b)

(c)

FIGURE 8.6   Keloid on right earlobe. (a) Before excision. (b) After excision. (c) Intralesional steroid injection immediately after excision.

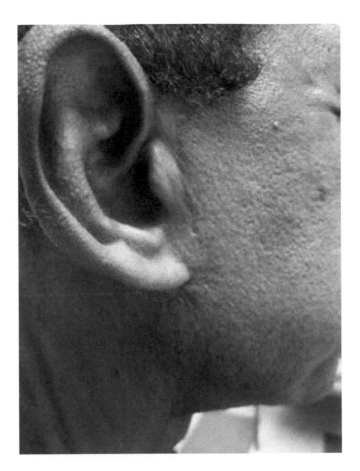

FIGURE 8.7   Well-healed scar after excision and intralesional steroid injections for a keloid.

It is also important to stop injecting areas where hypertrophy has resolved, as continued treatment may worsen a spread or depressed scar. This is a common mistake with novice injectors without a full understanding that this treatment is solely for the improvement of the thickened scar component.

Given their high efficacy for improving hypertrophic scars and keloids, injectable corticosteroids will continue to be a mainstay of treatment.

5-Fluorouracil

5-Fluorouracil (5-FU) is a pyrimidine antimetabolite, which has been used in the treatment of multiple malignancies and as an adjunct to glaucoma surgery. 5-FU has been shown to inhibit fibroblast proliferation *in vivo* and *in vitro*.[46] It also targets rapidly proliferating fibroblasts, blocks the TGF-β signaling pathway, and inhibits COL1A2 gene expression.[46]

In a study comparing the efficacy of intralesional corticosteroids, 5-FU, and combined therapy for the treatment of hypertrophic scars, the average onset of action was found to be similar for all three therapeutic modalities.[39] Transient burning sensation or discomfort was the

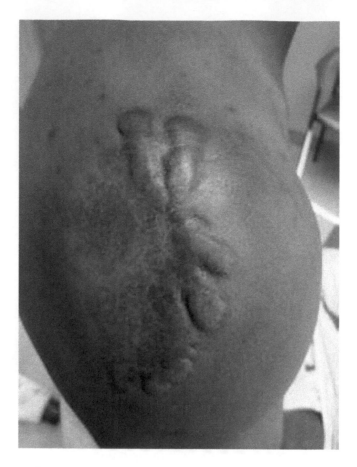

FIGURE 8.8   Excellent improvement in approximately one-half of a keloid after partial excision and intralesional steroid injections.

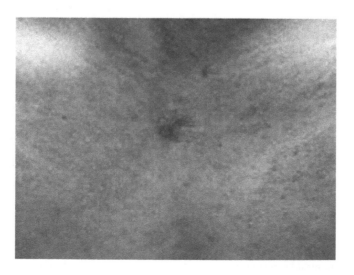

FIGURE 8.9   Minimal steroid-induced dermal atrophy in a partially treated keloid on chest.

most common side effect reported by patients in all groups. At week 32, the intralesional corticosteroid group began to demonstrate the sequelae of steroids, including atrophy, telangiectasia, and hypopigmentation, effects not noted in the 5-FU treatment arm. As for the primary outcomes, scar height, erythema, and pliability, 5-FU alone performed as well as steroids and the combination of steroids and 5-FU.[39] A separate investigation confirmed that the combination of intralesional corticosteroids and 5-FU is associated with fewer side effects than corticosteroids alone.[47] In a study of 50 keloids treated with topical silicone gel versus a combination of silicone and intralesional 5-FU injected immediately following excision, there was a statistically significant difference in the number of patients who were keloid-free at 1 year: 43% for the silicone group versus 75% for the combined therapy group.[48]

The most common regimen for intralesional injection of 5-FU is a concentration of 50 mg/mL, repeated every 1–2 weeks as needed. Alternatively, 0.1 mL of triamcinolone acetonide 40 mg/mL can be mixed with 5-FU and injected every 2 weeks. No local or topical anesthesia is needed prior to injection. The adverse effects associated with intralesional 5-FU are minimal and include local erythema, swelling, pain, dyspigmentation, and occasional ulcers.

In summary, a combination of intralesional 5-FU and corticosteroids appears to achieve better results than 5-FU alone and to decrease the adverse effects associated with corticosteroids. Thus, this combination may be an effective alternative for the treatment of recalcitrant hypertrophic scars and keloids.

Bleomycin

Bleomycin was isolated from a *Streptomyces verticillus* strain and found to have activity against neoplastic cells, bacteria, fungi, and viruses. It is used in the treatment of several malignancies and recalcitrant warts.[49,50] On the molecular level, bleomycin acts by binding to DNA, which leads to breaks in its structure.[44]

Bleomycin is known to cause keratinocyte necrosis, but its exact mechanism of action in scar reduction remains unclear. However, a possible explanation may be the inhibition of DNA synthesis by actively dividing fibroblasts in a dose-dependent manner.[51]

España et al. injected intralesional bleomycin into 13 keloids at a concentration of 1.5 IU/mL with a maximum dose of 2 mL/cm^2 or 6 mL per session.[52] The study demonstrated complete flattening (100%) in six cases, highly significant flattening (>90%) in six cases, and significant flattening (75%–90%) in the remaining case. In 2 of the 13 cases, a small nodule recurred approximately 1 year later. Aggarwal et al. used multiple superficial punctures to deliver bleomycin to 50 patients with keloids at intervals of 15 days for the first three applications, followed by a final application 2 months later.[53] The study found that 22 subjects (44%) had complete flattening and 11 (22%) had significant flattening of keloids. Regular follow-ups were performed for 18 months, and 7 subjects were found to have developed recurrences. The study also found that 40 subjects (88%) had complete relief of keloid-associated pruritus.

The adverse effects of intralesionally injected bleomycin are much less extensive and severe than those of systemic bleomycin, with the main ones being hyperpigmentation (75%)

and dermal atrophy (10%–30%). In addition, a case of flagellate hyperpigmentation after intralesional injection of bleomycin for verrucae plantaris has been documented.[54] On the other hand, the serious adverse effects associated with systemic administration, including hepatotoxicity and pulmonary fibrosis,[43] have not been reported to date with intralesional injections.

Preparation of bleomycin may be difficult in most outpatient settings because the medication must be reconstituted in a vertical laminar flow hood. Additionally, when handling the medication, nitrile gloves and eye protection are recommended. Nonetheless, bleomycin appears to be a promising treatment that should be further investigated.

EMERGING THERAPIES
Human Mesenchymal Stem Cells

Mesenchymal stem cells (MSCs) have the ability to differentiate into multiple cell types in response to specific local environments. MSC therapy has been reported in the treatment of cardiovascular disease, lung fibrosis, spinal cord injury, and bone and cartilage damage.[55-58] MSCs have been hypothesized to function as reservoirs of reparative cells and to be activated in response to wound signals or certain disease conditions. Several theories have been proposed to explain their role in wound repair, including the creation of a milieu that enhances regeneration of endogenous cells, differentiation, and transdifferentiation and angiogenesis.[59-61]

One study examined the role of transplanted human MSCs on wound healing in full-thickness cutaneous wounds in white rabbits.[62] A total of 15 white rabbits with 10 wounds per animal were examined. The study found that the transplanted MSCs significantly inhibited scar formation and increased wound tensile strength. In addition, MSCs from genetically unrelated donors did not elicit an immune response. MSCs represent an active area of research, and their role in human cutaneous wound repair needs to be examined in future studies.

Recombinant Human Transforming Growth Factor-β3

TGF-β has been studied as a potential scar-reducing agent since the 1980s, when it was discovered to play a major role in scar production. As discussed in Chapter 1, TGF-β is initially released by platelets at the site of injury and stimulates the migration of lymphocytes, fibroblasts, monocytes, and neutrophils. Levels of TGF-β are subsequently maintained by macrophages, fibroblasts, keratinocytes, and endothelial cells in the wound.[63,64]

Although TGF-β isoforms share a high degree of structural similarity, they each play a distinct role in the healing and scarring process. TGF-β1 and TGF-β2 have been shown to enhance extracellular matrix gene expression and to stimulate collagen and fibronectin synthesis by dermal fibroblasts, leading to tissue fibrosis.[62,63] In contrast, TGF-β3 has been found to reduce the influx of inflammatory cells, reducing subsequent scarring.[65] Additionally, adult wounds express higher levels of TGF-β1 and TGF-β2 than of TGF-β3 and are associated with scarring. Conversely, the relative levels are reversed in fetal wounds, which do not scar.[66] Thus, it has been hypothesized that wounds expressing TGF-β1 and TGF-β2 may lead to scar formation, while those expressing TGF-β3 may not.

Investigations into TGF-β as a scar-reducing agent have attempted to simulate the fetal wound-healing environment by increasing the ratio of TGF-β3 to TGF-β1 and TGF-β2. Lu et al. applied topical antibodies to TGF-β1, TGF-β2, and TGF-β3 to rabbit ear ulcers.[67] They found that wounds treated immediately after ulcer formation displayed delayed healing without scar reduction, while those treated 7 days after ulcer formation showed reduced scarring. Additionally, Shah et al. found that dermal wounds in rats treated with antibodies to TGF-β1 and TGF-β2 resembled normal dermis, in contrast to wounds in controls, which healed with scar formation.[68] They also found that treatment with an antibody to either TGF-β1 or TGF-β2 alone did not yield an improvement in scar formation, while exogenous TGF-β3 administration markedly reduced scarring.[69]

Avotermin is a human recombinant TGF-β3, which demonstrated significantly better scar appearance in double-blind placebo-controlled phase I and II studies,[70,71] but recently failed phase III studies. However, the amount of avotermin used in phase III trials was approximately one-half of that in phase II trials. All studies demonstrated a favorable safety profile without any adverse events reported. Although avotermin did not perform as expected in phase III trials, this will likely remain an active area of research.

Cyclooxygenase Inhibitors and Nonsteroidal Agents

As investigators have gained further knowledge of the role of the inflammatory cascade in scar formation, there has been an increased interest in the cyclooxygenase (COX) pathway. The two COX isoenzymes are COX-1 and COX-2; COX-1 mediates homeostatic functions, while COX-2 mediates the inflammatory pathway through prostaglandins and leukotrienes. Specifically, COX-2 catalyzes the conversion of arachidonic acid to prostaglandin E_2 (PGE_2), a major prostaglandin produced in the skin early in the inflammatory phase. PGE_2 is derived from keratinocytes within the epidermis and plays a role in keratinocyte differentiation, vascular permeability, and the activation and infiltration of inflammatory cells. Additionally, it has been shown that elevated levels of COX-2 can induce fibroblast proliferation and collagen production.[72] COX-1 and COX-2 are both inhibited by nonsteroidal agents (NSAIDs), such as aspirin and naproxen.

Using a topical COX-2 inhibitor on incisional wounds, Wilgus et al. were able to demonstrate a reduction in TGF-β1 and PGE2 levels during the inflammatory phase, which led to decreased collagen deposition and scarring.[73] Moreover, this was accomplished without disrupting reepithelization or decreasing tensile strength. Other researchers, however, have obtained conflicting results. For example, Blomme et al. found that a topical COX-2 inhibitor did not affect the healing of surgical skin wounds in a mouse model.[74]

Similarly, studies of the effect of additional inhibition of COX-1 have yielded contradictory results. A review by Su et al. found that NSAIDs may lead to excessive scar formation and delayed wound healing.[75] On the other hand, Muller-Decker et al. found that NSAIDs had no effect on tensile strength and did not delay wound healing.[76]

Given the important role of inflammation in scar formation and the low cost of NSAIDs, investigators will likely continue to pursue their potential as scar-reducing agents. However, since current studies show discordant results, additional investigations are needed at this time to fully evaluate their effects.

Angiotensin-Converting Enzyme Inhibitors

Angiotensin-converting enzyme (ACE) catalyzes the conversion of angiotensin I to angiotensin II and degrades bradykinin, a potent vasodilator. It is well accepted in the cardiology literature that ACE inhibitors play a critical role in down-regulating adverse fibrous cardiac remodeling.[77] Evidence of a renin-angiotensin system has also been demonstrated within human skin.[78] Additionally, elevated levels of ACE have been found in pathologic scar tissue compared to levels in normal and wounded skin.[79] Angiotensin II has also been shown to increase the production of type I collagen in dermal fibroblasts.[80]

One article documented the use of an ACE inhibitor for cutaneous wound healing. In it, Iannello et al. described two cases of keloids that were successfully treated with low-dose enalapril.[81] In one case, a keloid that developed after abdominal surgery was treated with 10 mg of enalapril for 4 months, with resultant complete resolution. In the second case, a 2-year-old keloid, also from abdominal surgery, was treated with the same dose of enalapril for 6 months, with subsequent marked improvement. These early promising results warrant further investigation into the role of ACE inhibitors in cutaneous scar reduction and remodeling.

Minocycline

Minocycline is a tetracycline antibiotic often used in the treatment of acne. It is also known to inhibit matrix metalloproteinases, which degrade the extracellular matrix.[82] A study by Henry et al. examined the effect of daily minocycline injections into standardized wounds on white rabbit ears for 4 weeks.[83] They found an 85% reduction in the mean hypertrophic index in the treated ear. While these findings are promising, research in humans may be impeded by the propensity of minocycline to cause pigment deposition in scars.

CONCLUSIONS

Numerous topical and injectable therapies exist for the treatment of postsurgical scars. While the evidence for some is strong, other agents, although popular, do not appear to offer any advantage beyond the normal wound healing process. Due to the high demand for scarless or nearly scarless cutaneous surgery, research in this field is very dynamic, with many new and promising agents being studied for this indication.

We have now come full circle, having started this book with a review of the molecular and cellular mechanisms of wound healing and ending with an examination of the potential impact of the new basic research findings on the development of future therapies. Combined with the best surgical techniques as discussed in previous chapters, a thorough understanding of the latest scientific developments in the field of wound healing will ensure that Mohs and dermatological surgeons stay at the forefront of cutaneous surgery and continue to deliver the best care for their patients and the most aesthetic postoperative results.

REFERENCES

1. Thomas JR, Somenek M. Scar revision review. *Arch Facial Plast Surg* 2012;14(3):162–74.
2. Reno F, Grazianetti P, Cannas M. Effects of mechanical compression on hypertrophic scars: Prostaglandin E_2 release. *Burns* 2001;27(3):215–8.
3. Chang LW, Deng WP, Yeong EK, Wu CY, Yeh SW. Pressure effects on the growth of human scar fibroblasts. *J Burn Care Res* 2008;29(5):835–41.
4. Van den Kerckhove E, Stappaerts K, Fieuws S, et al. The assessment of erythema and thickness on burn related scars during pressure garment therapy as a preventive measure for hypertrophic scarring. *Burns* 2005;31(6):696–702.
5. Ripper S, Renneberg B, Landmann C, Weigel G, Germann G. Adherence to pressure garment therapy in adult burn patients. *Burns* 2009;35(5):657–64.
6. Snyder GB. Button compression for keloids of the lobule. *Br J Plast Surg* 1974;27(2):186–7.
7. Chang CH, Song JY, Park JH, Seo SW. The efficacy of magnetic disks for the treatment of earlobe hypertrophic scar. *Ann Plast Surg* 2005;54(5):566–9.
8. Hassel JC, Roberg B, Kreuter A, Voigtländer V, Rammelsberg P, Hassel AJ. Treatment of ear keloids by compression, using a modified oyster-splint technique. *Dermatol Surg* 2007;33(2):208–12.
9. Hassel JC, Loser C, Koenen W, Kreuter A, Hassel AJ. Promising results from a pilot study on compression treatment of ear keloids. *J Cutan Med Surg* 2011;15(3):130–6.
10. Reiffel RS. Prevention of hypertrophic scars by long-term paper tape application. *Plast Reconstr Surg* 1995;96(7):1715–8.
11. Mustoe TA, Cooter RD, Gold MH, et al. International clinical recommendations on scar management. *Plast Reconstr Surg* 2002;110(2):560–71.
12. Mustoe TA. Evolution of silicone therapy and mechanism of action in scar management. *Aesthetic Plast Surg* 2008;32(1):82–92.
13. Hirshowitz B, Lindenbaum E, Har-Shai Y, Feitelberg L, Tendler M, Katz D. Static-electric field induction by a silicone cushion for the treatment of hypertrophic and keloid scars. *Plast Reconstr Surg* 1998;101(5):1173–83.
14. Hanasono MM, Lum J, Carroll LA, Mikulec AA, Koch RJ. The effect of silicone gel on basic fibroblast growth factor levels in fibroblast cell culture. *Arch Facial Plast Surg* 2004;6(2):88–93.
15. Kuhn MA, Moffit MR, Smith PD, et al. Silicone sheeting decreases fibroblast activity and downregulates TGFbeta2 in hypertrophic scar model. *Int J Surg Investig* 2001;2(6):467–74.
16. O'Brien L, Pandit A. Silicon gel sheeting for preventing and treating hypertrophic and keloid scars. *Cochrane Database Syst Rev* 2006;(1):CD003826.
17. Li-Tsang CW, Zheng YP, Lau JC. A randomized clinical trial to study the effect of silicone gel dressing and pressure therapy on posttraumatic hypertrophic scars. *J Burn Care Res* 2010; 31(3):448–57.
18. Carney SA, Cason CG, Gowar JP, et al. Cica-Care gel sheeting in the management of hypertrophic scarring. *Burns* 1994;20(2):163–7.
19. Hosnuter M, Payasli C, Isikdemir A, Tekerekoglu B. The effects of onion extract on hypertrophic and keloid scars. *J Wound Care* 2007;16(6):251–4.
20. Saulis AS, Mogford JH, Mustoe TA. Effect of Mederma on hypertrophic scarring in the rabbit ear model. *Plast Reconstr Surg* 2002;110(1):177–86.
21. Chung VQ, Kelley L, Marra D, Jiang SB. Onion extract gel versus petrolatum emollient on new surgical scars: Prospective double-blinded study. *Dermatol Surg* 2006;32(2):193–7.

22. Jackson BA, Shelton AJ. Pilot study evaluating topical onion extract as treatment for postsurgical scars. *Dermatol Surg* 1999;25(4):267–9.
23. Rashid SA, Halim AS, Muhammad NA. The effect of vitamin E on basic fibroblast growth factor level in human fibroblast cell culture. *Med J Malaysia* 2008;63 Suppl A:69–70.
24. Baumann LS, Spencer J. The effects of topical vitamin E on the cosmetic appearance of scars. *Dermatol Surg* 1999;25(4):311–5.
25. Jenkins M, Alexander JW, MacMillan BG, Waymack JP, Kopcha R. Failure of topical steroids and vitamin E to reduce postoperative scar formation following reconstructive surgery. *J Burn Care Rehabil* 1986;7(4):309–12.
26. Vissers WH, Berends M, Muys L, van Erp PE, de Jong EM, van de Kerkhof PC. The effect of the combination of calcipotriol and betamethasone dipropionate versus both monotherapies on epidermal proliferation, keratinization and T-cell subsets in chronic plaque psoriasis. *Exp Dermatol* 2004;13(2):106–12.
27. Takahashi H, Ibe M, Kinouchi M, Ishida-Yamamoto A, Hashimoto Y, Iizuka H. Similarly potent action of 1,25-dihydroxyvitamin D3 and its analogues, tacalcitol, calcipotriol, and maxacalcitol on normal human keratinocyte proliferation and differentiation. *J Dermatol Sci* 2003;31(1):21–8.
28. Bagot M, Charue D, Lescs MC, Pamphile RP, Revuz J. Immunosuppressive effects of 1,25-dihydroxyvitamin D3 and its analogue calcipotriol on epidermal cells. *Br J Dermatol* 1994;130(4):424–31.
29. van der Veer WM, Jacobs XE, Waardenburg IE, Ulrich MM, Niessen FB. Topical calcipotriol for preventive treatment of hypertrophic scars: A randomized, double-blind, placebo-controlled trial. *Arch Dermatol* 2009;145(11):1269–75.
30. Gudas LJ, Wagner JA. Retinoids regulate stem cell differentiation. *J Cell Physiol* 2011;226(2):322–30.
31. Otley CC, Gayner SM, Ahmed I, Moore EJ, Roenigk RK, Sherris DA. Preoperative and postoperative topical tretinoin on high-tension excisional wounds and full-thickness skin grafts in a porcine model: A pilot study. *Dermatol Surg* 1999;25(9):716–21.
32. Gunes Bilgili S, Calka O, Akdeniz N, Bayram I, Metin A. The effects of retinoids on secondary wound healing: Biometrical and histopathological study in rats. *J Dermatolog Treat* 2013;24(4):283–9.
33. Abdelmalek M, Spencer J. Retinoids and wound healing. *Dermatol Surg* 2006;32(10):1219–30.
34. Miller RL, Gerster JF, Owens ML, Slade HB, Tomai MA. Imiquimod applied topically: A novel immune response modifier and new class of drug. *Int J Immunopharmacol* 1999;21(1):1–14.
35. Berman B, Kaufman J. Pilot study of the effect of postoperative imiquimod 5% cream on the recurrence rate of excised keloids. *J Am Acad Dermatol* 2002;47 Suppl 4:S209–11.
36. Cacao FM, Tanaka V, Messina MC. Failure of imiquimod 5% cream to prevent recurrence of surgically excised trunk keloids. *Dermatol Surg* 2009;35(4):629–33.
37. Malhotra AK, Gupta S, Khaitan BK, Sharma VK. Imiquimod 5% cream for the prevention of recurrence after excision of presternal keloids. *Dermatology* 2007;215(1):63–5.
38. Sy GY, Nongonierma RB, Ngewou PW, et al. Healing activity of methanolic extract of the barks of *Spathodea campanulata* Beauv (Bignoniaceae) in rat experimental burn model. *Dakar Med* 2005;50(2):77–81.
39. Hong SS, Kim JH, Li H, Shim CK. Advanced formulation and pharmacological activity of hydrogel of the titrated extract of *C. asiatica*. *Arch Pharm Res* 2005;28(4):502–8.
40. Govindarajan R, Vijayakumar M, Rao CV, Shirwaikar A, Mehrotra S, Pushpangadan P. Healing potential of *Anogeissus latifolia* for dermal wounds in rats. *Acta Pharm* 2004;54(4):331–8.
41. Reish RG, Eriksson E. Scars: A review of emerging and currently available therapies. *Plast Reconstr Surg* 2008;122(4):1068–78.
42. Stojadinovic O, Lee B, Vouthounis C, et al. Novel genomic effects of glucocorticoids in epidermal keratinocytes: Inhibition of apoptosis, interferon-γ pathway, and wound healing along with promotion of terminal differentiation. *J Biol Chem* 2007;282(6):4021–34.
43. Diegelmann RF, Bryant CP, Cohen IK. Tissue alpha-globulins in keloid formation. *Plast Reconstr Surg* 1977;59(3):418–23.
44. Ardehali B, Nouraei SA, Van Dam H, Dex E, Wood S, Nduka C. Objective assessment of keloid scars with three-dimensional imaging: Quantifying response to intralesional steroid therapy. *Plast Reconstr Surg* 2007;119(2):556–61.

45. Manuskiatti W, Fitzpatrick RE. Treatment response of keloidal and hypertrophic sternotomy scars: Comparison among intralesional corticosteroid, 5-fluorouracil, and 585-nm flashlamp-pumped pulsed-dye laser treatments. *Arch Dermatol* 2002;138(9):1149–55.

46. Wendling J, Marchand A, Mauviel A, Verrecchia F. 5-Fluorouracil blocks transforming growth factor-β–induced α$_2$ type I collagen gene (*COL1A2*) expression in human fibroblasts via c-Jun NH$_2$-terminal kinase/activator protein-1 activation. *Mol Pharmacol* 2003;64(3):707–13.

47. Apikian M, Goodman G. Intralesional 5-fluorouracil in the treatment of keloid scars. *Australas J Dermatol* 2004;45(2):140–3.

48. Hatamipour E, Mehrabi S, Hatamipour M, Ghafarian Shirazi HR. Effects of combined intralesional 5-fluorouracil and topical silicone in prevention of keloids: A double blind randomized clinical trial study. *Acta Med Iran* 2011;49(3):127–30.

49. Froudarakis M, Hatzimichael E, Kyriazopoulou L, et al. Revisiting bleomycin from pathophysiology to safe clinical use. *Crit Rev Oncol Hematol* 2013;87(1):90–100.

50. Lewis TG, Nydorf ED. Intralesional bleomycin for warts: A review. *J Drugs Dermatol* 2006;5(6):499–504.

51. Hendricks T, Martens MF, Huyben CM, Wobbes T. Inhibition of basal and TGF beta-induced fibroblast collagen synthesis by antineoplastic agents. Implications for wound healing. *Br J Cancer* 1993;67(3):545–50.

52. España A, Solano T, Quintanilla E. Bleomycin in the treatment of keloids and hypertrophic scars by multiple needle punctures. *Dermatol Surg* 2001;27(1):23–7.

53. Aggarwal H, Saxena A, Lubana PS, Mathur RK, Jain DK. Treatment of keloids and hypertrophic scars using bleom. *J Cosmet Dermatol* 2008;7(1):43–9.

54. Abess A, Keel DM, Graham BS. Flagellate hyperpigmentation following intralesional bleomycin treatment of verruca plantaris. *Arch Dermatol* 2003;139(3):337–9.

55. Weil BR, Canty JM Jr. Stem cell stimulation of endogenous myocyte regeneration. *Clin Sci* (Lond) 2013;125(3):109–19.

56. Tzouvelekis A, Antoniadis A, Bouros D. Stem cell therapy in pulmonary fibrosis. *Curr Opin Pulm Med* 2011;17(5):368–73.

57. Vawda R, Fehlings MG. Mesenchymal cells in the treatment of spinal cord injury: Current and future perspectives. *Curr Stem Cell Res Ther* 2013;8(1):25–38.

58. Zarrabi M, Mousavi SH, Abroun S, Sadeghi B. Potential uses for cord blood mesenchymal stem cells. *Cell J* 2014;15(4):274–81.

59. Li H, Fu X. Mechanisms of action of mesenchymal stem cells in cutaneous wound repair and regeneration. *Cell Tissue Res* 2012;348(3):371–7.

60. Sasaki M, Abe R, Fujita Y, Ando S, Inokuma D, Shimizu H. Mesenchymal stem cells are recruited into wounded skin and contribute to wound repair by transdifferentiation into multiple skin cell type. *J Immunol* 2008;180(4):2581–7.

61. Wu Y, Chen L, Scott PG, Tredget EE. Mesenchymal stem cells enhance wound healing through differentiation and angiogenesis. *Stem Cells* 2007;25(10):2648–59.

62. Stoff A, Rivera AA, Sanjib Banerjee N, et al. Promotion of incisional wound repair by human mesenchymal stem cell transplantation. *Exp Dermatol* 2009;18(4):362–9.

63. Bullard KM, Longaker MT, Lorenz HP. Fetal wound healing: Current biology. *World J Surg* 2003;27(1):54–61.

64. Bettinger DA, Yager DR, Diegelmann RF, Cohen IK. The effect of TGF-beta on keloid fibroblast proliferation and collagen synthesis. *Plast Reconstr Surg* 1996;98(5):827–33.

65. Chang Z, Kishimoto Y, Hasan A, Welham NV. TGF-β3 modulates the inflammatory environment and reduces scar formation following vocal fold mucosal injury in rats. *Dis Model Mech* 2014;7(1):83–91.

66. Namazi MR, Fallahzadeh MK, Schwartz RA. Strategies for prevention of scars: What can we learn from fetal skin? *Int J Dermatol* 2011;50(1):85–93.

67. Lu L, Saulis AS, Liu WR, et al. The temporal effects of anti-TGF-β1, 2, and 3 monoclonal antibody on wound healing and hypertrophic scar formation. *J Am Coll Surg* 2005;201(3):391–7.

68. Shah M, Foreman DM, Ferguson MW. Control of scarring in adult wounds by neutralising antibody to transforming growth factor β. *Lancet* 1992;339(8787):213–4.

69. Shah M, Foreman DM, Ferguson MW. Neutralisation of TGF-beta 1 and TGF-beta 2 or exogenous addition of TGF-beta 3 to cutaneous rat wounds reduces scarring. *J Cell Sci* 1995;108(Pt 3):985–1002.

70. Ferguson MW, Duncan J, Bond J, et al. Prophylactic administration of avotermin for improvement of skin scarring: Three double-blind, placebo-controlled, phase I/II studies. *Lancet* 2009;373(9671):1264–74.

71. So K, McGrouther DA, Bush JA, et al. Avotermin for scar improvement following scar revision surgery: A randomized, double-blind, within-patient, placebo-controlled, phase II clinical trial. *Plast Reconstr Surg* 2011;128(1):163–72.

72. Wilgus TA, Bergdall VK, Tober KL, et al. The impact of cyclooxygenase-2 mediated inflammation on scarless fetal wound healing. *Am J Pathol* 2004;165(3):753–61.

73. Wilgus TA, Vodovotz Y, Vittadini E, Clubbs EA, Oberyszyn TM. Reduction of scar formation in full-thickness wounds with topical celecoxib treatment. *Wound Repair Regen* 2003;11(1):25–34.

74. Blomme EA, Chinn KS, Hardy MM, et al. Selective cyclooxygenase-2 inhibition does not affect the healing of cutaneous full-thickness incisional wounds in SKH-1 mice. *Br J Dermatol* 2003;148(2):211–23.

75. Su WH, Cheng MH, Lee WL, et al. Nonsteroidal anti-inflammatory drugs for wounds: Pain relief or excessive scar formation? *Mediators Inflamm* 2010;2010:413238.

76. Muller-Decker K, Hirschner W, Marks F, Furstenberger G. The effects of cyclooxygenase isozyme inhibition on incisional wound healing in mouse skin. *J Invest Dermatol* 2002;119(5):1189–95.

77. Rouillard AD, Holmes JW. Mechanical regulation of fibroblast migration and collagen remodelling in healing myocardial infarcts. *J Physiol* 2012;590(Pt 18):4585–602.

78. Steckelings UM, Wollschlager T, Peters J, Henz BM, Hermes B, Artuc M. Human skin: Source of and target organ for angiotensin II. *Exp Dermatol* 2004;13(3):148–54.

79. Morihara K, Takai S, Takenaka H, et al. Cutaneous tissue angiotensin-converting enzyme may participate in pathologic scar formation in human skin. *J Am Acad Dermatol* 2006;54(2):251–7.

80. Tang HT, Cheng DS, Jia YT, et al. Angiotensin II induces type I collagen gene expression in human dermal fibroblasts through an AP-1/TGF-β1-dependent pathway. *Biochem Biophys Res Commun* 2009;385(3):418–23.

81. Iannello S, Milazzo P, Bordonaro F, Belfiore F. Low-dose enalapril in the treatment of surgical cutaneous hypertrophic scar and keloid—two case reports and literature review. *MedGenMed* 2006;8(4):60.

82. Sapadin AN, Fleischmajer R. Tetracyclines: Nonantibiotic properties and their clinical implications. *J Am Acad Dermatol* 2006;54(2):258–65.

83. Henry SL, Concannon MJ, Kaplan PA, Diaz-Arias AA. The inhibitory effect of minocycline on hypertrophic scarring. *Plast Reconstr Surg* 2007;120(1):80–8.

INDEX

Milton Keynes UK
Ingram Content Group UK Ltd.
UKHW050451071024
449327UK00015B/328